Arsenic in Aquatic Environment

Arsenic in Aquatic Environment

Dr. S.P. Pande
Director-grade-Scientist (Retd.)
Project Advisor
Environmental Impact & Risk Assessment (EIRA) Division
NEERI, Nagpur – 440020 (M.S.)

Dr. Leena S. Deshpande
Sr. Technical Officer
Geo Environment Management (GEM) Division
NEERI, Nagpur – 440 020 (M.S.)

2010
DAYA PUBLISHING HOUSE
Delhi - 110 035

Published by   :   **Daya Publishing House**
                          A Division of
                          Astral International Pvt. Ltd.
                          – ISO 9001:2008 Certified Company –
                          4760-61/23, Ansari Road, Darya
                          Ganj, New Delhi-110 002
                          Ph. 011-43549197, 23278134
                          E-mail: info@astralint.com
                          Website: www.astralint.com

Laser Typesetting   :   **Classic Computer Services**
                          Delhi - 110 035

Printed at   :   **Chawla Offset Printers**
                          Delhi - 110 052

PRINTED IN INDIA

Foreword

Arsenic is ubiquitous element in nature and mainly transported in the environment through water. Humans may encounter arsenic in water from wells drilled into arsenic rich ground strata or from water contaminated by industrial or agrochemical wastes. In India, millions of persons in several districts of West Bengal, Uttar Pradesh, Bihar, Jharkhand, Assam, Chattisgarh and Punjab are drinking groundwater with arsenic concentrations far above acceptable level of 0.05 mg/L which is likely to be reduced to 0.01 mg/L in future. Thousands of people have already been diagnosed with poisoning symptoms, even though much of at-risk population has not yet been assessed for arsenic-related health problems. There are several organizations in the country, including the National Environmental Engineering Research Institute (NEERI), that are engaged in different R&D Projects related to arsenic management.

Efforts of Dr. Sunil P. Pande, Director-grade-Scientist (Retd.), NEERI and Dr. Leena S. Deshpande, Sr. Technical Officer, NEERI, in compiling the available arsenic related information and bringing it in the form of the book "*Arsenic in Aquatic Environment*" are gratefully appreciated. The book will serve as a useful reference material for all those who are engaged in researches towards the control of arsenic contamination in drinking water.

I hope this book will go a long way in providing valuable guidance to the environmental scientists/engineers in different parts of the globe, who are working towards providing arsenic-free drinking water to the affected population.

Dr. Tapan Chakrabarti
Acting Director
National Environmental Engineering Research Institute
Nehru Marg, Nagpur – 440 020

Preface

Arsenic is known as the king of poisons and had plagued human being since the days of antiquity. It is both a cause of large-scale environmental contamination and serious health hazard. Incidences of arsenic contamination in ground water and the subsequent sufferings of people from arsenic poisoning resulting from drinking arsenic contaminated water have been widely reported in the developed and developing countries. National Environmental Engineering Research Institute (NEERI) has been engaged in researches related to arsenic in drinking water since 1973. The groundwater pollution due to arsenic in the Chowki Block of Rajnandgaon District of Chattisgarh was reported for the first time by NEERI. A user-friendly field kit for arsenic has also been developed by NEERI on behalf of the World Health Organisation (WHO).

Besides NEERI there are several other organizations in India which are providing valuable R&D inputs towards solving the problem of arsenic in drinking water. However, there was a need to compile all the important achievements made under different projects related to arsenic and suitably document it so that it can form an easy reference material for the future generation researchers. In this backdrop, a thorough literature survey was made, information gathered from various R&D organizations, appropriate recommendations made, areas of further challenges delineated, and the documented material has been compiled in the form of this book *"Arsenic in Aquatic Environment"*. Special reference has been made in this book to the recommendations of WHO, which has contributed significantly in providing financial, technical and man-power support to resolve this global environmental menace of arsenic in groundwater.

The literature provided by different R&D organizations for preparing a Base Paper on Arsenic under a sponsored project of Rajiv Gandhi National Drinking Water Mission (RGNDWM), Ministry of Rural Areas & Employment, Government of India has contributed significantly towards the preparation of this book. We convey our sincere thanks to all the devoted project leaders whose valuable R&D contributions are included in this book. We are extremely thankful to Dr. S.R. Wate, Director-grade-Scientist, and Head, EIRA Division, NEERI, Nagpur for his constant encouragement and valuable support in the preparation of this book.

We hope that this book will go a long way in providing valuable guidance to all the research workers who are engaged in de-arsenification studies of groundwater.

Dr. S.P. Pande
Dr. Leena S. Deshpande

Contents

List of Figures

List of Tables

Chapter 1
Introduction

Arsenic is a group VA metalloid, with atomic number 33 and atomic weight 74.9216. As a group V element, arsenic exhibits a broad range of chemical reactivity with an ability to form alloys with other elements, and covalent bonds with carbon, hydrogen and oxygen. It is also known to readily participate in oxidation-reduction, methylation-demethylation and acid-base reactions.

Water is one of the major means of transport of arsenic in the environment. Arsenic in aquatic environment is predominant in places with high geothermal activities. Soil erosion and leaching have been reported by MacKenzie et al.[1] to contribute to 612 and 2380 × 10^8 g/yr. of arsenic in the dissolved and suspended form to the oceans. Soil erosion and agricultural runoff are large contributors to the arsenic concentration in sediments. High arsenic levels (8.6–13.2 mg/g) have been reported by Viraraghavan et al.[2] to be associated with sediments and a potential exists that it may be released in hazardous amounts to the overlying waters. Industrial effluents are a major source of arsenic in the environment. Arsenic and arsenical compounds are found in effluents from metallurgical industry, glassware and ceramic industry, dye and pesticide manufacturing industry, petroleum refining, rare earth industry and other organic and inorganic chemical industries. It finds application in the manufacture of herbicides and pesticides. Other industries using arsenic include wood and hide preservative; lead shot manufacture; phosphate detergent builder and presoaks used in many fertilizers[3]. With the development of organic arsenic compounds, many of the inorganic arsenic compounds have declined in use. Arsenic is a cause for skin, liver, lung, and kidney/bladder cancer. Due to the carcinogenic property of arsenic, regulatory agencies are reviewing its maximum allowable concentration levels in drinking water.

Chapter 2
Occurrence of Arsenic in the Environment

2.1 Rocks, Soils, and Sediments

Arsenic is widely distributed in a large number of minerals. The highest mineral concentrations generally occur as arsenides of copper, lead, silver, or gold or as the sulfide. Major arsenic-containing minerals are arsenopyrite (FeAsS), realgar (As_4S_4), and orpiment (As_2S_3). The arsenic content of the earth's crust is 1.5–2 mg/kg; it ranks 20th in abundance in relation to other elements. Oxidized forms of arsenic are usually found in sedimentary deposits. The elemental oxidation state, though stable in reducing environments, is rarely found. Table 1 gives some ranges of arsenic contents in different rocks. Although the values shown are generally low, mineralized zones of sulfidic ores may contain much higher concentrations of arsenic.

Table 1: Arsenic Concentration in Rocks

Type of Rock	Arsenic (mg/kg)
Igneous	
Ultrabasic	
Periodotite, dunite, serpentinite	0.3–15.8
Basic	
Basalts (extrusive)	0.18–113
Gabbro (intrusive)	0.06–28
Intermediate	
Latite, andesite, trachyte (extrusive)	0.5–5.8
Diorite, granodiorite, syenite (intrusive)	0.09–13.4
Acidic	
Rhyolite (extrusive)	3.2–5.4
Granite (intrusive)	0.18–15
Metamorphic rocks[5]	
Quarzite	2.2–7.6
Slate/phyllite	0.5–143
Schist/gneiss	0.0–18.5
Sedimentary rocks[6,7,8]	
Marine	
Shale/claystone (nearshore)	4.0–25
Shale/claystone (offshore)	3.0–490
Carbonates	0.1–20.1
Phosphorites	0.4–188
Sandstone	0.6–9
Nonmarine	
Shales	3.0–12
Clay stone	3.0–10

Source: From Welch, A.H., Lico, M.S., and Hughes, J.L., Ground Water, 26(3), 333, 1988.

High levels of arsenic may also occur in some coals. The average arsenic content of coal in the USA was estimated at 1–10 mg/kg[9]. In some coal mined in Czechoslovakia, the concentration of arsenic has been shown to be as high as 1500 mg/kg.[10]

Uncontaminated soils were found to contain arsenic levels between 0.2 and 40 mg/kg, while arsenic-treated soils contained up to 550 mg/kg[11]. The soil in the city of Antofagasta, Chile, contains natural levels of arsenic of about 3.2 mg/kg.[12] In the Comarca Lagunera, Mexico, values between 3 and 9 mg/kg were found at the soil surface and more than 20 mg/kg, deep down[13].

Peat may contain considerable quantities of arsenic. Minkkinen and Yliruokanen[14] found maximum arsenic concentrations in various Finnish peat bogs of between 16 and 340 mg/kg dry peat.

The natural level of arsenic in sediments is usually below 10 mg/kg dry weight[15]. Bottom sediments can become substantially contaminated by arsenic from man-made sources. Levels of up to 10000 mg/kg dry weight were found in bottom sediments near a copper smelter in Washington, USA[15].

2.2 Air

Airborne particulate matter has been shown to contain both inorganic and organic arsenic compounds.[16, 17] Crecelius[15] showed that only 35 per cent of the inorganic arsenic in rain from an urban area was present as arsenite; however, some post-sampling oxidation could not be excluded. In studies by Johnson and Braman,[16] methylarsines made up approximately 20 per cent of the total arsenic in ambient air from rural and urban areas.

In unpolluted areas, airborne arsenic concentrations ranging from less than one to a few nanograms per cubic metre have been reported.[18, 19, 16, 20, 21]

2.3 Water

Arsenic occurs in both inorganic and organic forms in water[22, 15]. The main organic arsenic species, methylarsonic acid and dimethylarsinic acid, are generally present in smaller amounts than the inorganic forms, arsenite and arsenate. The chemistry of arsenic in the aqueous environment has been reviewed by Ferguson and Gavis[23].

The arsenic contents of surface waters in unpolluted areas vary but typical values seem to be a few micrograms per litre or less. In a study of river waters in the USA, about 80 per cent of the samples contained levels of less than 0.01 mg/litre[24]. Quentin and Winkler[25] found an average value of 0.003 mg/litre in river water and 0.004 mg/litre in lake water in the Federal Republic of Germany. A mean arsenic concentration of 0.0025 mg/litre was reported in some Norwegian rivers[26]. Much higher values have been reported[27] from some areas including Antofagasta, Chile, where the average arsenic level in a river water supply of drinking water between 1958 and 1970 was 0.8 mg/litre.

The oxidation state of arsenic in surface waters in various parts of the world remains largely unknown. Braman and Foreback[22] found that the ratio of trivalent to pentavalent inorganic arsenic ranged from <0.06 to 6.7 in a few uncontaminated surface water samples containing between 0.0025 and 0.0030 mg As/litre. About 8 per cent of the total arsenic in 2 samples of well-aerated stream water (0.014 and 0.06 mg/litre, respectively) was reported by

Clement and Faust[28] to be in the trivalent form. In anaerobic reservoirs, all of the arsenic present (0.14–1.3 mg As/litre) seemed to be in this form.

Penrose *et al.*[29] reported that sea-water ordinarily contains arsenic concentrations ranging from 0.001–0.008 mg/litre. Levels of about 0.002 mg/litre have been reported by Onishi[30] and Johnson and Braman[31]. The major chemical form of arsenic appears to be the thermodynamically stable arsenate ion; even so, arsenite often accounts for one third of the total arsenic[32,33].

Clement and Faust[28] analysed water from 2 groundwater supplies with very high levels of arsenic (224 and 280 mg/litre) and found that about 50 per cent was present as arsenic(III). In a groundwater fed stream, 26 per cent of the total arsenic (0.08 mg/litre) was in the form of trivalent arsenic. Arsenic speciation has also been performed on well water samples from an area in Alaska containing high levels of arsenic[34]. In 5 samples containing arsenic concentrations ranging from 0.52 to 3.6 mg/litre, between 3 per cent and 39 per cent of the arsenic present was trivalent, the rest being pentavalent. No methylated arsenic compounds could be detected.

High levels of arsenic have been found in waters from areas of thermal activity. Thermal waters in New Zealand have been shown to contain up to 8.5 mg/litre.[35] Geothermal water in Japan contained arsenic levels of 1.8–6.4 mg/litre and neighbouring streams contained about 0.002 mg/litre[36].

The chemical forms of arsenic in thermal water from New Zealand were investigated by Aggett and Aspell[37]. In the geo-thermal bores, more than 90 per cent of the arsenic was present in the trivalent form. However, in a river flowing through the area, the pentavalent form was predominant but some seasonal variation in the ratio between the two valence states was indicated.

Arsenic in groundwater has been found above the maximum permissible limit (0.05 mg/L) in six districts of West Bengal, India; these six districts have an area of 34,000 km^2 with a population of 30 million[38,39]. It was estimated, based on a survey of small areas of the arsenic affected districts in West Bengal, that at least 800.000 people could be drinking water high in arsenic with more than 175,000 people showing arsenical skin lesions that are the late stages of manifestation of arsenic toxicity. The source of arsenic is geological. Most of the water samples contained a mixture of arsenite and arsenate and in none of them, methylarsonic or dimethylarsinic acid was detected.

A study of groundwater samples collected in an area of about 270 km^2 from Chennai City, India showed that the arsenic levels exceeded the maximum permissible limit over the entire city and a positive correlation of arsenic with other toxic metals showed that all these toxic elements are anthropogenic in origin[40].

Arsenic contamination of well waters in Nova Scotia, Canada was first identified in 1976 when a resident of Waverly (Halifax county) was diagnosed as being intoxicated with arsenic. The well water in the resident's home was found to contain 0.5 mg/L of arsenic, which was ten times the maximum acceptable concentration in Canada of 0.05 mg/L. A follow up study of 198 wells in the Waverly area indicated that 34 wells were contaminated with arsenic above the maximum permissible limit[41]. A survey of ground water supplies in Halifax county revealed consistent MCL violations in various communities[42]. In at least 10 per cent of the samples analyzed, the arsenic contamination was in excess of 500 µg/L while, 23 per cent of the samples analysed were found to contain arsenic higher than 250 µg/L[42].

2.4 Biota

The sorption of arsenate ions in the soil by iron and aluminum components, greatly restricts the availability of arsenic to plants[43]. The arsenic content of plants grown on soils that had never been treated with arsenic-containing pesticides varied from 0.01 to about 5 mg/kg dry weight[4]. Plants grown on arsenic-contaminated soils may, however, contain considerably higher levels, especially in the roots[44,11,45]. Some grasses growing on soils containing high levels of arsenic have been found to have elevated arsenic contents[46]. Anderson and Nilsson[47] reported that arsenic in soils treated with sewage sludge was highly available to plants, but only a few samples were analysed. In contrast, Furr *et al.*[48] claimed that soil arsenic is not readily available to plants.

Marine algae and seaweed usually contain considerable amounts of arsenic. Lunde[49] showed values of '10–100 mg/ kg dry weight in marine algae from the Norwegian coast. The degree of enrichment was found to be between 1500 and 5000 compared with the level of arsenic in the growth medium[50]. Similar and even higher enrichment ratios were reported for fresh water plants in the Waikato River, New Zealand[51]. The elevated arsenic concentrations in the water (0.03–0.07 mg/litre) gave rise to concentrations of up to 971 mg As/kg dry weight in aquatic plants.

Chapter 3
Cases of Arsenic Poisoning and Arsenic Toxicity

Arsenic has acquired an unparalleled reputation as a poison, with arsenic trioxide, a tasteless and odorless inorganic arsenic compound, constituting a convenient agent for homicide[52]. High levels of arsenic (0.9 to 3.4 mg/ L) in well waters in the Cordoba region of Argentina was responsible for 165 deaths. A high proportion of deaths was due to cancer of the respiratory system and gastrointestinal tract[52]. High arsenic levels have also been found in the water supplies in Chile and Ghana. The toxicity of arsenic is dependent on its oxidation state, chemical form and solubility in the biological media[53]. The toxicity of As(III) is about ten times that of As(V)[54]. An acute high dose of arsenic by oral intake causes gastrointestinal irritation resulting in difficulty in swallowing, thirst, abnormally low blood pressure and convulsions. The lethal dose for adults has been noted to be 1-4 mg As/kg[54].

A study on cancer risks from arsenic in drinking water indicates that arsenic could cause liver, lung, kidney/ bladder cancer other than skin cancer[55]. The study showed that the lifetime risk of dying from cancer of the liver, lung, kidney or bladder on consumption of 1L/day of water containing 50µg/L of arsenic could be high as 13 per 1000 persons. In the United States, over 350,000 people may be drinking water containing more than 50 µg/L of arsenic and over 2.5 million people could be supplied with water having arsenic levels over 25 µg/L. Based on the average arsenic levels and water consumption patterns in the United States, the risk was estimated to be around 1 per 1000.

A survey of 114 wells in Tainan region of the south west coast of Taiwan showed arsenic concentrations ranging from 0.6 to 2.0 mg/L[56]. Blackfoot disease, a peripheral disorder characterized by gangrene of the extremities, especially the foot, was the cause of 244 deaths. A chemical factory manufacturing several chemicals including the insecticide Paris–Green (acetocopper arsenite), was responsible for the contamination of wells in the southern part of Kolkata, India[57]. Over seven thousand people were consuming the arsenic contaminated water for several years, but this fact remained unnoticed until September 1989. A few died, and some of the victims were hospitalized, while symptoms of arsenic poisoning were evident in many families living in the area. Water samples analysed for arsenic indicated extremely high levels of contamination, with total arsenic concentration ranging from as low as 0.002 to as high as 58 mg/L.

In 1984, two projects for improving the quality of the drinking water for 100,000 people were completed in the Xinjiang Uighur Autonomous Region of China, an area of endemic arsenic toxicosis[58]. A follow-up study of the area showed that an improvement in the symptoms and signs of arsenic poisoning in humans occurred as a result of the new drinking water sources indicating that the disease can be controlled by supplying arsenic-free water in areas of endemic arsenic toxicosis[58].

A survey conducted by the American Water Works Association (AWWA) for inorganic contaminants in water supplies in the United States revealed 34 violations for arsenic (maximum contaminant level (MCL) 0.05 mg/L), with concentration values ranging from 0.052 to 0.190 mg/ L and a mean concentration of 0.083 mg/L[59]. A combined AWWA-USEPA data base revealed 46 MCL violations. Most of the violations were reported in New Mexico, Texas and Oklahoma. Isolated cases of arsenic violations occurred in Alaska, North Carolina, New Hampshire, Virginia and Illinois. A summary of the worldwide arsenic problem including that in West Bengal and Bangladesh is given at Annexure VIII.

3.1 Toxicity of Arsenic

Exposure

Human exposure to inorganic arsenic may occur through inhalation and ingestion. Inhalation usually occurs occupationally or during cigarette smoking. In unpolluted areas the amount of arsenic inhaled per day is about 0.05 mg or less. Depending on the content of arsenic in tobacco, an average smoker may inhale between a few micrograms and 20 μg of arsenic daily. Occupational exposure to arsenic may occur among smelter workers and workers exposed in the production and use of arsenic containing pesticides. In most food stuffs arsenic mainly occurs in the organic form and concentrations are usually less than 1 mg/kg. However, marine fish may contain arsenic upto 5 mg/kg. The total daily intake of arsenic by the general population is usually less than 0.2 mg/day, but is greatly influenced by amount of seafood in the diet. Exposure to arsenic through ingestion occurs mainly by drinking contaminated water. Drinking water ordinarily may contain a few micrograms of arsenic per litre. Levels exceeding maximum permissible limit (50 µg/L) in water may lead to health effects.

Mechanism

Arsenic is not a physiological constituent of the body. Absorption, excretion and retention of arsenic in the human body is influenced by the amount and the chemical forms in which it is ingested. Arsenic in the forms that is ordinarily present in food and the organic compounds of arsenic acid, are well absorbed. Following absorption arsenic is distributed rapidly and widely to all tissues of the body e.g. liver, kidney, spleen, heart, jejunum, marrow, lungs, pancreas, muscles, stomach, thyroid, skin, brain and spinal cord. In the body trivalent arsenic is oxidized to pentavalent state. The opposite can also take place. Inorganic arsenic is methylated to organic form dimethyl arsenic acid and mono methyl arsonic acid. The methylation of inorganic arsenic in the body is a detoxification process, which reduces the affinity of the compounds for the tissues. The arsenic (III) in the body combines with sulphydryl containing substances and inhibits the activity of many enzymes of the group. It interferes with cell enzymes, cell respiration and mitosis.

The excessive arsenic intake can lead to health/physical problems in the body of the consumers of arsenic affected drinks and food. Other than ingestion arsenic causes toxicity through inhalation. Arsenic affects all the organs and systems of the body. The toxicity of arsenic compounds depends on the chemical and physical form of the compound, the route by which it enters the body, the dose and the duration of exposure, dietary levels of interacting elements and the age and sex of the exposed individuals. Arsenite (III) is more toxic than Arsenate (V). Arsenic in solution is more toxic than undissolved arsenic. The toxicity of arsenic decreases in the order : Arsine > Inorganic Arsenic (III) > Organic Arsenic (III) > Inorganic Arsenic (V) > Organic Arsenic (V) > Arsonium Compounds and elemental arsenic.

Excretion

Both trivalent and pentavalent inorganic arsenic in solution are readily absorbed after ingestion. When arsenic is absorbed into the body, the major portion is excreted mainly through urine and a small portion through faeces. Arsenic is also eliminated through skin, hair, and nail and to some extent through bronchial secretions. After administration arsenic appears in urine within 2 to 8 hours. About 25 per cent being excreted in 24 hours and about 75 per cent within 7 days of exposure. The major metabolites found in the urine are methyl arsonic acid and dimethylarsinic acid. A portion of the absorbed arsenic is deposited in the skin, hair and nails where it is firmly bound to keratin. Storage in these metabolically 'dead' tissues is responsible for the slow elimination rate of arsenic. Arsenic in urine, hair and nails has thus been used as an index for monitoring the exposure of victim to arsenic and urinary arsenic is generally reported as the most reliable indicator of recent exposure to inorganic arsenic. Blood arsenic is not considered a good indicator because it is cleared within a few hours of absorption. In unexposed persons arsenic concentration in urine range from 0.01–0.05 mg/litre, in hair usually below 1 mg/kg and in blood 0.0015–0.0025 mg/litre.

3.2 Clinical Manifestation

Arsenic can give rise to acute and chronic toxicity in the body. Acute toxicity occurs only from the ingestion of arsenic compounds. The symptoms of acute toxicity include: severe vomiting and diarrhea, muscular cramp, facial oedema and cardiac abnormalities. An ingested dose of 70-180 mg of arsenic (III) oxide has been reported to be fatal in man. Symptoms of acute toxicity may occur within a few minutes of exposure if the arsenic compound is in solution but may be delayed for several hours if it is solid or taken with a meal.

The clinical manifestations due to chronic arsenic toxicity develop very insidiously after six months to two years or more depending on the amount of arsenic intake. Chronic toxicity of arsenic is best discussed in terms of the organ systems affected–the skin, nervous system, liver, cardiovascular system, and respiratory tract.

Effects on Skin

A number of skin lesions have been attributed to chronic exposure to inorganic arsenic compounds. Symmetric hyperkeratosis of the palms and soles is a characteristic finding after long-term ingestion of inorganic arsenic in drinking water or drugs. Approximately 1mg of arsenic intake per day for several years may give rise to skin effects. Hyper pigmentation (melanosis) of the skin, often associated with paler spots (depigmentation), is commonly encountered and occurs mainly in the areas of the skin not exposed to the sun, *i.e.,* axillae and trunk. Melanosis is also observed in tongue and buccal mucus membrane. Other than Bangladesh these lesions have been reported from regions in Argentina, Chile, Taiwan, Japan, Mexico and India where the contents of arsenic in drinking water were elevated.

Liver Toxicity

The chronic absorption of arsenic occasionally produces hepatocellular toxicity, which may be the result of an inhibition of arsenic by the enzymes, involved in cellular respiration. Trivalent arsenic binds readily to sulfhydryl groups of enzymes and has been shown to inhibit pyruvate dehydrogenase function that alternation has been correlated with swelling and distortion of the hepatic mitochondrias. Chronic exposure to arsenic has been reported to produce reversible liver enlargement and has been associated with cirrhosis of the liver. Nonchirrhotic portal hypertension has also been reported following chronic arsenic intake.

Cardiovascular Toxicity

Peripheral vascular disease has been observed among persons in Chile and in Taiwan who had chronic exposure to arsenic in drinking water. Early symptoms included acrocyanosis and Raynaud's phenomenon. Those changes were associated with hyper pigmentation and hyperkeratosis. These progressed in severe cases to frank gangrene of the extremities (blackfoot disease) associated with endarteritis obiliterans. In Chile, infants and children showed more pronounced vascular symptoms than adults, and myocardial infarction was reported even in children.

Neurologic Toxicity

Peripheral neuropathy affecting primarily sensory function has been encountered in several studies of persons with chronic exposure to arsenic. The prevalence of sensory and motor symptoms correlated positively with the concentration of arsenic in well water as well as with the arsenic content in hair. Possible hearing loss reflecting arsenic toxicity to the eighth cranial nerve was reported in a study.

Haemopoietic Toxicity

Chronic exposure to arsenic has been associated with disturbed erythropoiesis, and megaloblastic formation has been noted. These changes may reflect the inhibitory effects of arsenic on cellular respiration. Depression of delta aminolevulinic acid synthetase and of ferrochelatase activity in experimental animals dosed with arsenic has been reported.

Respiratory Toxicity

In early stages of arsenic intoxication respiratory infection is found to be associated with other clinical manifestations. Lung cancer has been found among the people exposed to arsenic trioxide.

Endocrine Toxicity

Diabetis Mellitus and Goiter have also been reported in association with prolonged ingestion of arsenic through drinking water.

Carcinogenicity

Available epidemiological and toxicological data indicate that arsenic is a toxic chemical and carcinogen in man. Arsenic has been found to cause cancer of the skin, liver, lung, urinary bladder, prostate, and possibly of haemopoietic and lymphatic tissues. Inorganic arsenic have indicated an association with lung cancer.

Operational Definitions

Melanosis

Blackening/darkening of skin diffuse or spotted due to deposition of black pigment (melanine) in the skin and mucous membrane due to stimulation of melanocyte.

(a) Mild–blackening of skin (melanosis), thinly distributed in palm, trunk, gum, tongue, lips etc. (both spotted and diffuse)

(b) Moderate–melanosis densely affecting gum, palm and trunk (spotted and diffuse) with leucomelanosis (rain drop pigmentation).

(c) Severe–melanosis densely and extensively affected gum, palm, trunk and whole body with leucomelanosis.

Leucomelanosis

Depigmentation in hyper pigmented area characterised by whitish /pallor patch in rain drop manner, due to exhaust melanocyte.

Keratosis

Rough, dry, hard, and thickening of epithelium due to increased keratinization, keratosis is palpable and in most cases distribution is symmetric.

(*a*) Mild–Just palpable keratosis (spotted and diffuse) but not clearly visible scatteringly affecting palm and sole.

(*b*) Moderate–Palpable and visible keratosis (spotted and diffuse) affecting palm and sole

(*c*) Severe–Wart like keratosis (spotted and diffuse) hands, legs and feet.

Hyper Keratosis

Densely and extensively distributed keratosis affecting whole palm and sole.

Some typical cases of melanosis of trunk and the palm, and keratosis of the sole and the palm are depicted in Plates 1 and 2.

The cutaneous effects including skin cancers of chronic exposure to high levels of arsenic in drinking water have been demonstrated by epidemiological studies of exposed populations in South America, Taiwan, India, Argentina and Mexico.

Arsenic exposure has been associated with three types of skin cancers–Bowen's disease, Basal cell carcinoma, and Squamous cell carcinoma; these cancers are frequently multiple in origin and develop primarily from arsenical keratoses. The prevalence of arsenic-related skin cancer appears to depend upon total absorbed dose of arsenic. A total of about 20 gm arsenic over a lifetime resulted in a prevalence of skin cancer of about 6 per cent.

Clinical Feature

Sign and symptoms of chronic arsenicosis differ in manifestations in different countries. The clinical manifestations are categorised in the following stages.

Pre Clinical Stage

☆ Not detectable by clinical manifestation

Initial Stage

☆ Melanosis (spotted, diffuse)

☆ Keratosis (spotted, diffuse)

☆ Conjunctivitis

☆ Bronchitis

☆ Gastroenteritis

Second Stage

☆ Depigmentation (leucomelanosis – rain drop pigmentation)

☆ Hyperkeratosis

☆ Oedema of legs (non pitting)

☆ Peripheral neuropathy

☆ Nephropathy (early stage)

☆ Hepatopathy (early stage)

Last Stage

☆ Nephropathy (late stage)

☆ Hepatopathy (late stage)

☆ Gangrene

☆ Cancer (skin, bladder and lung)

3.3 Treatment and Management

So far there is no specific treatment for chronic arsenicosis.

Withdrawal of further intake of arsenic contaminated water and taking arsenic free water, improve the cases. Chelation therapy and vitamins and nutritious diet enhance the recovery.

Chelation Therapy

Recently chelation therapy for the treatment of arsenicosis is considered to be specific therapy for relief of systemic clinical manifestations and reduction of arsenic stores in the body, decreasing subsequent cancer risk. The chelating agents which are currently recommended for the treatment of chronic arsenicosis are:

δ-Penicillamine

Dose: 250 mg 3 to 4 times a day for 3 months δ-Pencillamine is a costly drug and in 20 to 30 per cent cases may develop toxic effects. These include skin rash, fever, thrombocytopenia and leucopenia. Rare side effects include auto-immune haemolytic anaemia and stevens–Johnson Syndrome, anorixia, nausea, sleep disturbance, urinary frequency and nephrotoxicity may be seen occassionally. Patient receiving penicillamine should be carefully monitored for these side effects by observing manifestations and blood examination.

DMSA (dimercapto succinic acid) 10 mg/kg body weight for first 7 days, followed by 10 mg/kg thrice daily for 14 days.

DMPS (dimercapto propane sulphonate) 100 mg 3 to 4 times a day for every alternate week upto 3 courses.

Nutritious Diet and Vitamins

Symptoms are improved by good diet and vitamins. High protein diet help in the clearance of inorganic arsenic by increased methylation and protects against toxic effect of arsenic. The antioxidants vitamins, A, E, and C play an important role for management of cases. Vitamin C reduces the toxicity of arsenic and deficiency of vitamin A increases sensitivity to arsenic. These vitamins may be given to the arsenicosis patient in the following doses for 3 months.

Vitamin A–50, 000 i.u daily for adult

Vitamin E–200 mg daily

Vitamin C–500 mg daily

In case of children reduced dose should be given.

Excessive intake of vitamin A more than 1,00, 000 I.U daily for months may produce chronic toxicity in the body such as appetite loss, dry skin, bone and joint pain, enlarged liver and spleen, abnormal skin pigmentation. Acute toxicity of Vitamin A may develop if more than 3,00,000 I.U is taken at a time. Vitamin E is relatively non-toxic. Adults appear to be able to tolerate dose as high as 1000 I.U per day. Excessive dose of vitamin C, 2 gm or more may produce side effects.

People should be advised to take more protein and vitamin rich food like beans, peas, pulse, lentils, wheat, soyabean, green and leafy vegetables.

Other Symptomatic Treatment

Keratosis of palm and sole can be treated by local application of keratolytic ointment–20 per cent urea and 10 per cent to 20 per cent salicylic acid in cream or vaseline. Cryosurgery can also be done to remove keratosis. Treatment of associated fungal infection with ointment and medicine also improve the cases.

Chapter 4
Evidence of Arsenic Essentiality

Studies with minipigs, goats, chicks, hamsters, and rats have indicated that arsenic is an essential nutrient[60,61]. Currently, there is insufficient data for the assessment of arsenic essentiality in humans; therefore, conclusive evidence of human essentiality is lacking[62]. As a result, the Food and Nutrition Board[63] of the National Research Council and USEPA[64] do not consider arsenic to be an essential element for humans.

The potential nutritional requirement for humans has been calculated. The safe and adequate daily dietary intake for humans must be extrapolated from animal studies, and an intake of' 12 to 40 µg has been suggested for adults[62,65]. Uthus[65] has noted that no human pathological condition has been attributed to arsenic deprivation, but this may be because arsenic is typically present in the diet.

Recently, Mayer *et al.*[66] reported a positive correlation between lowered arsenic serum levels in hemodialysis patients and central nervous system injury, cancer, and vascular diseases. They concluded that "arsenic should be considered or may be defined to be essential for human life processes." Additional studies are needed, however, to firmly establish the essentiality of arsenic in humans.

Chapter 5

Guideline Limits for Arsenic in Drinking Water

Due to the carcinogenicity of some arsenic compounds, the objective should be to reduce its exposure to a level as close to zero as possible, taking into consideration its health effects and toxicology, occurrence and human exposure, availability and cost of the treatment technology, the practical quantitation limit of analytical techniques and the estimated risk for cancer at the low concentrations of arsenic normally found in drinking water. Based on these considerations, some regulatory agencies have revised the maximum contaminant level for arsenic in drinking water. An interim maximum acceptable concentration (IMAC) value of 25 µg/L has been established in Canada[67]. The

U.S. Environmental Protection Agency had initially considered lowering the arsenic MCL from the existing 50 µg/L to between 10 and 20 µg/L[68]. A further downward revision of the MCL to a range between 2 and 20 µg/L is being considered[69]. Table 2 indicates the guideline values for arsenic drinking water supplies by various regulatory agencies[70,71]. Even though the toxicity of arsenic is largely dependent on its chemical form, the guideline values target only the total arsenic concentration.

Table 2: Guideline Values for Arsenic Established by Various Regulatory Agencies[70,71]

Country/Organization	Maximum Contaminant Level (MCL) µg/L
Canada	25 (IMAC)
USA	50*
France	50
Federal Republic of Germany	40**
World Health Organization (WHO)	50
European Economic Community (EEC)	50
India	50[40]
China	50[58]
Taiwan	50[58]

*: USEPA was considering downward revision to 2–20 µg/L[69]

**: This was proposed to be lowered to 10 µg/L in 1996[72]

5.1 Provisional Guideline Value (WHO Guidelines for Drinking Water Quality, 1996)

Inorganic arsenic compounds are classified by International Agency for Research on Cancer (of WHO) in Group 1 (carcinogenic to humans) on the basis of sufficient evidence for carcinogenicity in humans and limited evidence for carcinogenicity in animals[73]. No adequate data on the carcinogenicity of organic arsenicals is available. The guideline value has been derived on the basis of estimated lifetime cancer risk.

Data on the association between internal cancers and ingestion of arsenic in drinking water is limited and insufficient for quantitative assessment of an exposure-response relationship[74]. However, based on the increased incidence of skin cancer observed in the population in China (Province of Taiwan), the US Environmental Protection Agency has used a multistage model that is both linear and quadratic in dose to estimate the lifetime skin cancer risk associated with the ingestion of arsenic in drinking-water. With this model and data on males[74], the concentrations of arsenic in drinking-water associated with estimated excess lifetime skin cancer risks of 10^{-4}, 10^{-5}, and 10^{-6} are 1.7, 0.17, and 0.017 µg/litre, respectively.

It should be noted, however, that these values may overestimate the actual risk of skin cancer because of possible simultaneous exposure to other compounds in water and possible dose-dependent variations in metabolism that could not be taken into consideration. In addition, the concentration of arsenic in drinking-water at an estimated skin cancer risk of 10^{-5} is below the practical quantification limit of 10 µg/litre.

A value of 13 µg/litre may be derived (assuming a 20 per cent allocation to drinking-water) on the basis of the provisional maximum tolerable daily intake (PMTDI) of inorganic arsenic of 2 µg/kg of body weight set by the Joint FAO/WHO Expert Committee on Food Additives (JECFA) in 1983 and confirmed as a provisional tolerable weekly intake (PTWI) of 15 µg/kg of body weight in 1988[75]. JECFA noted, however, that the margin between the PTWI and intakes reported to have toxic effects in epidemiological studies was narrow.

With a view to reducing the concentration of arsenic in drinking-water, a provisional guideline value of 0.01 µg/litre is recommended by WHO. The estimated excess life-time risk of skin cancer associated with exposure to this concentration is 6×10^{-4}. It is important to note that this provisional guideline value of 0.01 mg/litre is for total arsenic. No guideline value has been suggested so far for arsenate or arsenite in drinking water.

Chapter 6

Environmental Chemistry of Arsenic

Arsenic generally exists in the inorganic form in water supplies. Under different redox conditions, arsenic is stable in the +5, +3, –3 and 0 oxidation states. The pentavalent (+5) or arsenate species are AsO_4^{-3}, $HAsO_4^{-2}$, and $H_2AsO_4^{-}$. The trivalent (+3) or the arsenite species include $As(OH)_3$, $As(OH)_4^{-}$, AsO_2OH^{-2} and AsO_3^{-3}. The pentavalent arsenic species are predominant and stable in the oxygen-rich aerobic environments, whereas, the trivalent arsenite species are predominant in moderately reducing anaerobic environment such as groundwater[76]. The pH determines the predominant arsenate or arsenite species. The stability and the predominance of the arsenic species in aquatic environments at different pH ranges is shown in Table 3[77].

Table 3: Stability and Predominance of Arsenic Species in Varying pH Ranges in the Aquatic Environment

pH	0–9	10–12	13	14
As (III)	H_3AsO_3	$H_2AsO_3^-$	$H_3AsO_3^{2-}$	AsO_3^{3-}
pH	0–2	3–6	7–11	12–14
As(V)	H_3AsO_4	$H_2AsO_4^-$	$H_3AsO_3^{2-}$	AsO_4^{3-}

Arsenic in its soluble form generally occurs in its +3 and +5 oxidation states.' Both, organic and inorganic forms of arsenic can be detected in natural water systems. Methylated or organic arsenic occurs at concentrations less than 1 µg/L and is not of major significance in drinking water treatment[78]. Arsenic in its various chemical forms and oxidation states is released into the aquatic environment by natural erosion processes and industrial discharges. On release to the aquatic environment, the arsenic species enter into a methylation/demethylation cycle, while some are bound to the sediments or taken up by biota where they could undergo metabolic conversion to other organo arsenicals[79]. Several fungi and bacterial species have been demonstrated to methylate inorganic arsenic by an initial reduction to arsenite, and the addition of methyl groups[79]:

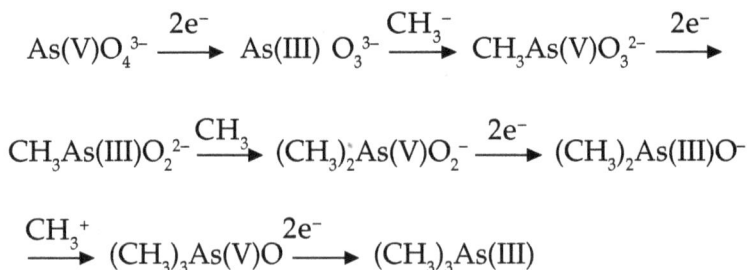

$$As(V)O_4^{3-} \xrightarrow{2e^-} As(III)\ O_3^{3-} \xrightarrow{CH_3^-} CH_3As(V)O_3^{2-} \xrightarrow{2e^-}$$

$$CH_3As(III)O_2^{2-} \xrightarrow{CH_3} (CH_3)_2As(V)O_2^- \xrightarrow{2e^-} (CH_3)_2As(III)O^-$$

$$\xrightarrow{CH_3^+} (CH_3)_3As(V)O \xrightarrow{2e^-} (CH_3)_3As(III)$$

Chapter 7

Transformation of Arsenic Species

Little is known about the rate of oxidation of As(III) to As(V) in natural waters.[80] The rate of oxidation of As(III) to As (V) is reported to be very slow at neutral pH values, but proceeds measurably in several days in strongly alkaline or acid solutions[81]. No quantitative information, however, is available on aerobic surface waters[82]. However, some authors have reported that the oxidation reaction occurs quickly and that environmental samples must be analyzed within a few hours of collection or significant amounts of As(III) will be converted to As(V)[83, 84]. This rapid oxidation, however, was not detected in soil extracts containing 5 to 500 µ/L of As(III)[85].

In summary, the rate of reduction of As(V) or oxidation of As (III) cannot be predicted based on a few simple measurements. The effects of microorganisms, the effects of solid surfaces, and how these effects vary with temperature, pH, and Eh have not been described. It is probably not possible to determine rates of reaction until the nature of these other relationships is fully understood.

Organisms affect the distribution of arsenic by accumulating,[86] transporting,[87] and transforming[88] it. Bacteria and marine phytoplankton can reduce As (V) to As (III) or catalyze the oxidation of As(III) to As(V)[89]. Biological reduction of As (V) reportedly occurs most easily when the pH is between 6 and 6.7. The *eq* for the reaction is between 77 and 167 mV[90]. Thus, the relative concentration of As (V) and As (III) may be affected by the

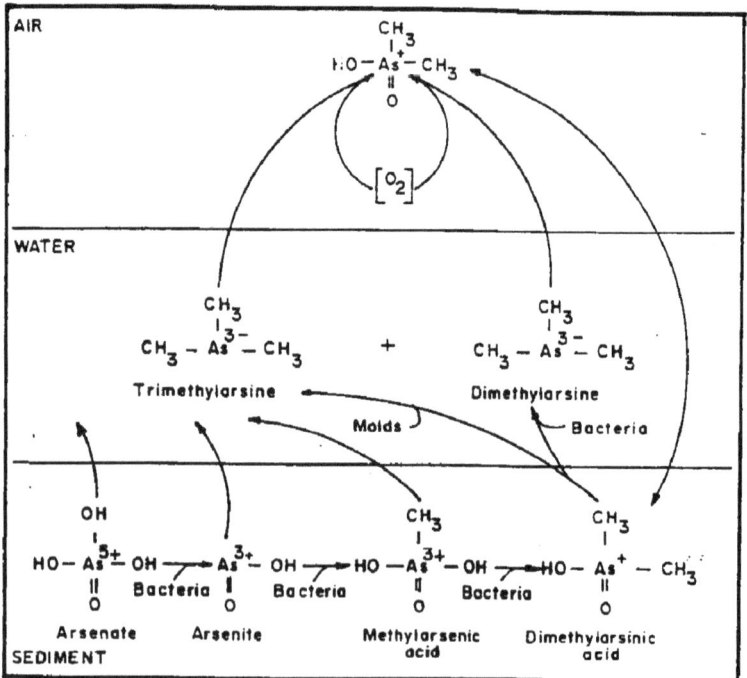

Figure 1: The Biological Cycle for Arsenic

bacterial populations[91]. The extent and impact of the biological reactions is debatable.

Some of the transformations, such as oxidation of As(III) to As(V) are probably catalyzed by organisms such as methanogenic bacteria,[92] but also occur in their absence.[82] The latter authors report, however, that As (III) is not completely oxidized to As (V) in natural waters unless microorganisms catalyze the reaction. At the same time, others have stated that microbial oxidation of As(III) was unimportant.[84, 93] A biological cycle for arsenic has been postulated by Wood,[94] as shown in Figure 1. The figure demonstrates that microorganisms are believed capable of reducing As (III) to mono- and dimethyl arsenic acids and arsines. Such reactions, however, are not completely understood.[91]

Chapter 8
Mechanism for Arsenic Occurrence in Groundwater

It is reported that the occurrence of As(III) in groundwater may be more widespread than is generally assumed[95]. The circumstances reported by Matisoff et al.[96] and Korte[97] are probably more common than previously suspected. A suggested mechanism for the appearance of As(III) is presented conceptually in Figure 2. In Figure 2A, As (V) is retained in stream sediments in adsorption reactions. This mechanism is consistent with the work of Livesay and Huang,[98] who demonstrated that arsenic retention, at low arsenic concentrations, does not proceed through the precipitation of sparingly soluble As(V) compounds, but rather through adsorption mechanisms.

Moreover, the adsorption maxima are linearly related to the content of sesquioxides and clay. Indeed, recent studies involving acid mine drainage have demonstrated that the dissolved concentration of arsenic is regulated by sorptive processes with iron oxyhydroxides.[99, 100] Other researchers have also reported that arsenic partitions into iron-rich phases in soils and sediments.[101, 102, 103]

An important aspect of the accumulation phase is that adsorption equilibrium is reached within minutes while desorption is slow,[104] demonstrating that arsenic will continue to accumulate in a stream bed so long as the sesquioxides continue to accumulate. Indeed, under certain circumstances, adsorption may be irreversible,[105] indicating that only a change in Eh and the concomitant alteration of the oxide structure will result in release of the arsenic.

Figure 2B shows that once the arsenic-bearing sediments are buried and subjected to reducing conditions, the iron and manganese oxides are reduced and the arsenic is reduced and mobilized. This release into the groundwater is similar to releases from reducing sediments, as recently reported by Moore *et al.*[106] who showed that reduction causes the iron and manganese to dissolve. The only difference is that in Moore's study there was ample sulfide which resulted in the precipitation of As(III) sulfides rather than the mobilization of free As(III).

An example involving groundwater is shown in Figure 3. This well log was obtained from an alluvial system in central Ohio. A new well was drilled because an older adjacent well, that was fully screened in the saturated zone, contained arsenic exceeding the U.S. drinking water standard of 0.05 mg/l. The old well had been in use for

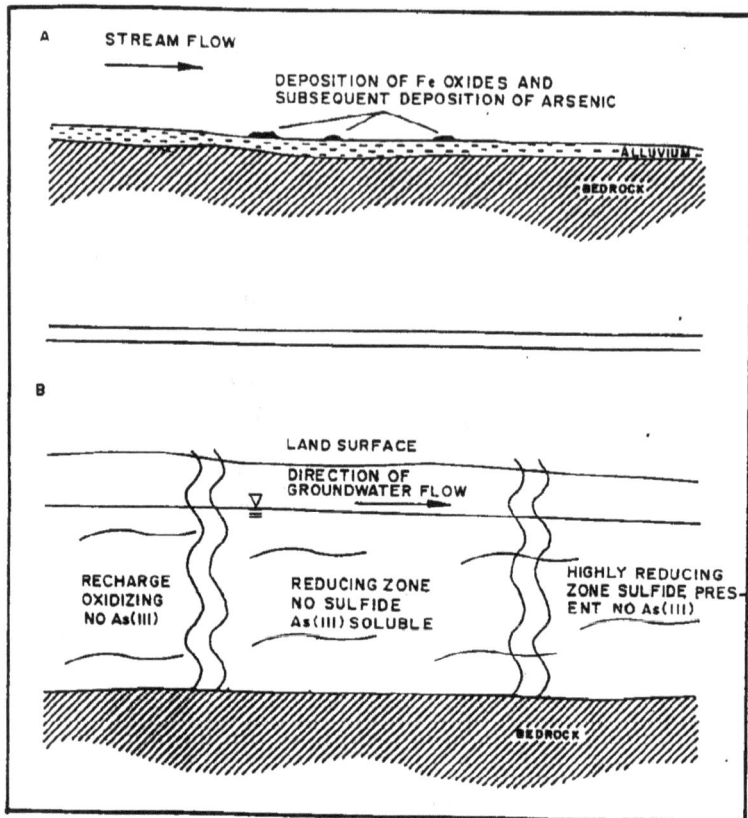

**Figure 2: (A) Conceptual Diagram Showing the Deposition
of Arsenic with Fe Oxides in a Surface Water System;
(B) Conceptual Diagram Showing the Dissolution of
As(III) following Burial of the Alluvium and the
Onset of Reducing Conditions**

many years but had only recently been sampled for arsenic.
Figure 3 shows the existence of a reduced iron and arsenic-
rich zone. The new well was screened above this zone and
no arsenic was detected (detection limit was 0.01 mg/l) in
the new water supply.

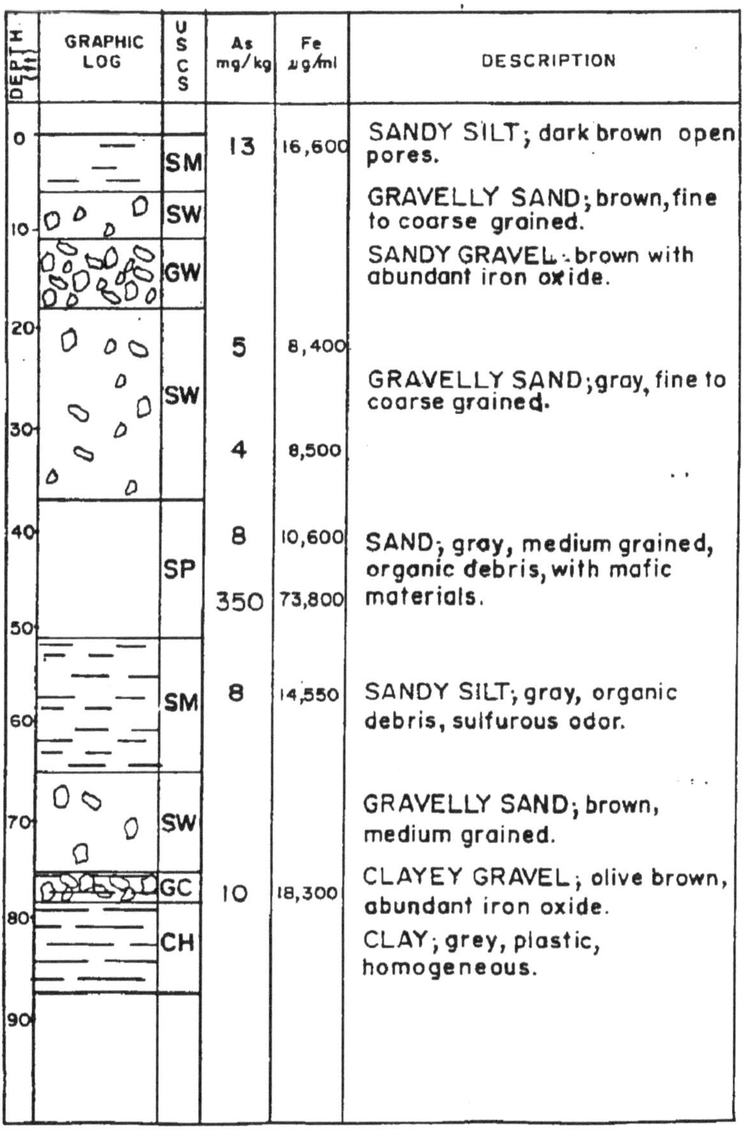

DEPTH (ft)	GRAPHIC LOG	U S C S	As mg/kg	Fe µg/ml	DESCRIPTION
0		SM	13	16,600	SANDY SILT; dark brown open pores.
10		SW			GRAVELLY SAND; brown, fine to coarse grained.
		GW			SANDY GRAVEL - brown with abundant iron oxide.
20			5	8,400	
30		SW	4	8,500	GRAVELLY SAND; gray, fine to coarse grained.
40		SP	8	10,600	SAND; gray, medium grained, organic debris, with mafic materials.
50			350	73,800	
60		SM	8	14,550	SANDY SILT; gray, organic debris, sulfurous odor.
70		SW			GRAVELLY SAND; brown, medium grained.
80		GC	10	18,300	CLAYEY GRAVEL; olive brown, abundant iron oxide.
		CH			CLAY; grey, plastic, homogeneous.
90					

**Figure 3: Well Log from Ohio Showing
Reduced Iron/Arsenic Zone**

Chapter 9
Methods of Arsenic Analysis

The 20th Edition (1998) of Standard Methods for the Examination of Water and Wastewater (Prepared and published jointly by American Public Health Association, American Water Works Association and Water Environment Federation) has recommended three methods for the analysis of arsenic in drinking water samples. These are (A) Atomic Absorption Spectrometric method, (B) Silver Diethyldithiocarbamate (SDDC) method and (C) Inductively Coupled Plasma method.

Unpolluted fresh water normally does not contain organic arsenic compounds, but may contain inorganic arsenic compounds in the form of arsenate and arsenite. The studies carried out in India by Mandal et al.[107] has also shown that organic form of arsenic is absent in the groundwaters in the seven districts of West Bengal surveyed by them. The hydride generation–atomic absorption method (A), which converts arsenic compounds to their hydrides that subsequently are decomposed in an argon-hydrogen flame, is the method of choice, although the electro-thermal method (direct injection of sample into the graphite tube) is a simpler method in the absence of interferences in the water sample.

The silver diethyl dithiocarbamate (SDDC) method (B), in which arsine is generated by sodium borohydride in acidic solution, is applicable to the determination of total inorganic arsenic when interferences are absent and the sample contains no methyl arsenic compounds. Because arsenite is more toxic than arsenate, a method for identification of these two species has been developed using SDDC method.

The inductively coupled plasma (ICP) method (C) is useful at higher concentrations (greater than 50 µg/L) of arsenic. However, if hydride generation technique is coupled with ICP method then the sensitivity can be increased manifolds.

Standard Method for Arsenite and Arsenate Determination in Drinking Water

Arsenite, containing trivalent arsenic, is reduced selectively by aqueous sodium borohydride solution to arsine, AsH_3, in an aqueous medium of pH 6. Arsenate, methylarsonic acid, and dimethyl arsenic acid are not reduced under these conditions. The generated arsine is swept by a stream of oxygen-free nitrogen from the reaction vessel through a scrubber containing glass wool or cotton impregnated with lead acetate solution into an absorber tube containing SDDC and morpholine dissolved in chloroform. A red colour-develops, the intensity of which is measured at 520 nm. To determine total inorganic arsenic in the absence of methylarsenic compounds, reduce another sample portion at a pH about 1. Alternatively, arsenate can be determined in a sample from which arsenite has been removed by reduction at pH 6, after acidification with hydrochloric acid and addition of another portion of sodium borohydride solution. The arsine formed from arsenate is collected in fresh absorber solution.

Some of the earlier work on the analysis of arsenic in drinking water was carried out in this country by Pande *et al.* [108, 109, 110–114] using the silver diethydithiocarbonate method. This method was further improved by Chakraborty *et al.*[115] Recently a flow injection-hydride generation-atomic absorption spectrometry (FI-HG-AAS) has been developed at the School of Environmental Sciences, Jadavpur University, by Chakraborty *et al.*[116, 117] for the analysis of arsenic in water, urine, and digested hair, nail and skin-scale samples.

Although a large number of analytical methods have been developed, by different researchers for the estimation of arsenic in water samples, they have not yet been allotted the status of Standard Method as per the guidelines of the Standard Methods Committee. A more detailed account of sample preservation and analysis of arsenic is given under Annexures I and II, which includes methods for total arsenic, analysis for specific arsenic compounds, and recent developments in the determination of arsenic species in water samples.

Chapter 10
Technologies for Arsenic Removal from Drinking Water

Many small communities are faced with arsenic contamination of their groundwater supplies at levels higher than the MCL specified by the various regulatory agencies. A survey for arsenic in surface water and groundwater systems showed higher levels in groundwater systems.[54] Groundwater systems showed arsenic concentrations ranging from <0.5 µg/L–38.6 µg/L with an average arsenic concentration of 2.4 µg/L. The surface water systems showed a arsenic concentration range of <0.5 µg/L–4.6 µg/L, with a average concentration of 0.6 µg/L.[69] Utilities having a blend of surface/groundwater showed an arsenic concentration range between <0.5 µg/L–4.6 µg/L and a average of 1.5 µg/L. A community being supplied with water containing an inorganic contaminant higher than MCL have two possible solutions: change to a new water source; or incorporate treatment methods either at the point-of-entry or at the point-of-use treatment to meet the contaminant MCL.[118, 119] In many cases, treatment of the source water may be the only option available.

Various treatment methods have been adopted to remove arsenic from drinking water under both laboratory and field conditions. The major mode of sequestering arsenic from water is by physical-chemical treatment methods. The various treatment methods include:

☆ Adsorption-co-precipitation using iron and aluminum salts;

☆ Adsorption on activated alumina/activated carbon/activated bauxites;

☆ Reverse osmosis;

☆ Ion exchange; and

☆ Oxidation followed by filtration.

The United States Environmental Protection Agency (USEPA) has summarized coagulation with iron and aluminum salts, and lime softening as the most effective treatment process for removing arsenic from water to meet the interim primary drinking water regulations standard of 0.05 mg/L.[120] Oxidation of As(III) Co As(V) and removal using the above processes has been recommended. Jekel in a recent review also concluded that if As (III) is present in a water source, oxidation must be applied, followed by the precipitation of As V by ferric salts.[72]

10.1 Coagulation

Coagulation is one of the most conventional processes used for the removal of arsenic from water. Table 4 presents a summary of arsenic removal by coagulation.

USEPA has shown that >90 per cent removals of arsenic (0.3 mg/L) can be achieved by application of alum at pH < 7, ferric chloride at pH < 8.5 or by lime softening at pH > 10.5.[120] Iron and alum coagulation methods were studied for the removal of 0.1 to 20 mg/L As(V) from water samples.[121,122] River water, well water and tap water were spiked to achieve the above As(V) concentrations used in the laboratory studies. As(V) removals were found to depend on its initial concentration. Thus, at As (V) concentrations <1.0 mg/L, coagulation with 30 mg/L of either alum or ferric sulfate resulted in > 90 per cent removals.[123] At As (V) concentration >1.0 mg/L, ferric sulphate was found to perform better than aluminum sulfate. For example, removal of 2 mg/L of As(V) with 30 mg/L of ferric sulfate and 100 mg/L of aluminum sulfate, was found to be comparable (>90 per cent). Also at 20 mg/L As (V), ferric sulfate was more effective than alum. As(V) removals were found to improve with an increase in pH.

More than 90 per cent removal of 0.05 mg/L As(V) was achieved at pH of 5.0–7.0 using 30 mg/L of either ferric sulfate or alum.[133] Ferric sulfate performed better than alum above pH 7.0. Ferric sulfate coagulation achieved higher removals (40–60 per cent) for As (III) compared to alum (5–15 per cent).

Aluminum and ferric hydroxide have been used to remove 0.05 mg/L As(V) from solution.[134] Ferric hydroxide was found to be more effective for As(V) removal compared

Table 4: Arsenic Removal by Coagulation

Arsenic Species	Treatment Method	Coagulant Dosage (mg/L)	Initial Conc. (mg/L)	Removal (Per cent)	pH	Reference
As(V)	FeCl$_3$	5	0.050	100	7.0	78
As(III)	FeC$_3$	6	0.005	72	8.0	78
As(III)	FeCl$_3$	18	0.005	84	8.0	78
*	Aeration, alum coagulation, settling and 6 days filtration	7	0.8	70	7.4	56
*	Aeration, FeCl$_3$ coagulation, settling and 10 days filtration	18.5	0.69	60	7.4	56
*	Aeration, alum coagulation, settling and 12 days filtration	21	0.70	46	7.4	56
*	Chlorine (20mg/L) oxidation, aeration. FeCl$_3$ coagulation, settling and 20 days filtration	51	0.83	100	7	56
*	FeCl$_3$	30	1	92	6.8	56
As (V)	Ferric chloride	20	0.045	96	7.5	124
As (V)	Ferric chloride	40	0.045	95	7.5	124
As (V)	Ferric chloride	40	0.043	97	8	124

Contd...

Table 4—Contd...

Arsenic Species	Treatment Method	Coagulant Dosage (mg/L)	Initial Conc. (mg/L)	Removal (Per cent)	pH	Reference
As (V)	Alum	60	0.043	97	8	124
As (V)	Alum coagulation	30	<1-2	≥ 90	6.4-7.5	121
As (V)	Ferric sulfate coagulation	30	<1/2	> 90	6.4-7.5	121
AS(III), As(V) and methane arsonate	Ferric chloride	*	30-40	90-95	5.5	125
As (V)	Alum	>5	0.2	97.5	7	126
As (V)	Ferric sulfate	5	0.2	97.5	7	126
As (V)	Hydrous manganese oxide	20	0.2	76	7	126
AS(III)	Ferric chloride	200	31	86	10	127
As(III)	Ferric chloride	500	31	92	10	127
As(III)	Ferric chloride	1000	31	93	10	127
As (V)	Electrochemical iron addition, hydrogen peroxide oxidation, settling and filtration	*	56	99.8	6.5	128

Contd...

Table 4—Contd...

Arsenic Species	Treatment Method	Coagulant Dosage (mg/L)	Initial Conc. (mg/L)	Removal (Per cent)	pH	Reference
As (III)	Ferric sulfate coagulation	10	0.2	62	7.5	129
As (III)	Ferric sulfate coagulation	10	0.2	75	7.5	129
As (III)	$FeCl_3$	10	0.2	76	7.5	129
As (III)	Cupric sulfate coagulation	10	0.2	88	7.5	129
As (III)	Cuprous chloride coagulation	10	0.2	85	7.5	129
As (III)	Zinc chloride coagulation	10	0.2	84	7.5	129
As (III)	$FeCl_3.6H_2O$	300	100	78	8	130, 131
As (III)	Ag_2SO_4	625	100	82	8	130, 131
As (III)	$CuSO_4.5H_2O$	300	100	85	8	130, 131
As (III)	$Al_2SO_4.18H_2O$	300	100	73	8	130, 131
*	$KMnO_4$ (13.8 mg/L) oxidation, ferric sulfate coagulation and filtration	28	0.7	86	7.4	132

*: Information or data not given by the authors.

to aluminum hydroxide. Table 5 shows As(V) removal as a function of pH and coagulant dose.

Table 5: As(V) Removal as a Function of pH and Coagulant Dose[134]

Initial pH	Dosage of Alum, and Iron (mg/L)	As(V) Removal (per cent) by Alum after Sedimentation and Filtration	As(V) Removal (per cent) by Iron after Sedimentation and Filtration
5.0	10	59	97
	20	82	97
	30	91	96
	40	93	95
	50	92	99
6.0	10	75	97
	20	89	98
	30	91	98
	40	89	>99
	50	94	98
7.0	10	65	94
	20	82	97
	30	84	97
	40	91	>99
	50	92	98
8.0	10	19	89
	20	39	90
	30	47	97
	40	67	96
	50	66	97

Note: Initial As(V) conc. 0.05 mg/L.

Ferric hydroxide as a complexing precipitant was found to be the most efficient and cost effective method for the removal of inorganic arsenic and methyl arsonate from subsurface leachate and groundwater.[125] Laboratory studies indicated that the addition of ferric chloride at an iron to arsenic ratio of 7 to 1, adjusting pH to 5.5 and settling overnight, achieved 90–95 per cent reduction in 30 to 40 mg/L initial arsenic concentration. A polyeletrolyte was added to enhance flocculation and settling. Arsenic concentration of 30 mg/L was reduced to 0.7 mg/L. The cost of treatment was given as $0.02 per gallon treated, with a range of $0.01 to $0.10 per gallon treated.

Lauf and others have studied the removal of As (III) and As(V) by ferric sulfate and hydrous manganese oxide (HMO).[126] Isotherm studies using jar test indicated poor As (III) removal by the adsorbents as compared to As(V). The isotherms for the adsorption of As(V) and As(III) were developed by varying the concentration of the adsorbents. The concentration of As(III) or As(V) was maintained at 200 µg/L and the pH of the solution was 7.0. Alum showed no removal for As(III) upto alum dosage of 25 mg/L. However, above alum dosages of 5 mg/L, the adsorption of As(V) was found to be 97.5 per cent. Based on the studies, an alum dosage of 25 mg/L was calculated for the removal of 1 mg/L of As(V). A pH range from 6 to 7 was suggested as an optimum pH range for the removal of As (V) from solution by 20 mg/L of alum. Ferric sulfate showed high removal for As(V). As(V) removal of 97.5 per cent was achieved at ferric sulfate dosage of 5mg/L at pH 8. A pH range between 4 to 8 was suggested as the optimum pH range for the removal of As(V) from solution by 10 mg/L of ferric sulfate. HMO formed *in situ* gave higher arsenic removals. The freshly formed HMO removed <10 per cent As(III). HMO was formed in situ by oxidizing Mn(II) with

$KMnO_4$ in the As(III)/As(V) solution. This *in situ* formation of HMO was believed to aid in arsenic removal by adsorption and coprecipitation. The removal of arsenic by HMO was not affected by pH, and an initial concentration of 200 μg/L was reduced to 48 μg/L. The adsorption data was represented by the Langmuir and Freundlich isotherms. The $KMnO_4$ demand for oxidizing As(III) to As(V) was given as 1.26 mg/L $KMnO_4$ per mg/L As(III). The oxidation reaction was found to be independent of pH in the range between 6 and 8.

Batch studies indicated ferric.chloride as the most effective coagulant when compared to hydrated lime, sodium sulfide or alum.[127] Ferric chloride dosages of 200, 500 and 1000 mg/L reduced an initial As(III) concentration of 31 mg/L to 4.3, 2.4 and 2.1 mg/L at pH 10, respectively, indicating removals of 86 per cent, 92 per cent and 93 per cent. Arsenic was effectively removed using electrochemical iron addition, chemical oxidation using hydrogen peroxide, settling and filtration from contaminated wastewater.[128] An influent arsenic concentration of 56 mg/l was reduced to 0.095 mg/L (99.8 per cent removal) using the above process at a pH of 6.5. The arsenic removal goal at the site was 0.19 mg/L. Based on bench scale and pilot plant studies, an iron to arsenic ratio of 5:1 was suggested for optimum arsenic removal.

Ferric chloride was found to be the most effective coagulant for the removal of arsenic from water.[56] An initial arsenic concentration of 1 mg/L in the raw water having a pH of 6.8 was reduced to 0.08 mg/L (92 per cent removal) using 30 mg/L dosage of $FeCl_3$. Oxidation with chlorine followed by ferric chloride coagulation resulted in effluent arsenic levels lower than 0.05 mg/L. Addition of 15 mg/L of chlorine followed by coagulation with 30 mg/L of $FeCl_3$ reduced arsenic (0.8 mg/L) concentration to trace amounts in the treated water. Pilot scale studies were conducted using raw water from contaminated wells containing 0.8 to 0.9 mg/L arsenic. Addition of about 20 mg/L of chlorine during the aeration process followed by $FeCl_3$ (about 60 mg/L) coagulation, settling and filtration resulted in an effluent with arsenic below the detection limit. Based on the outcome of experimental results, a full scale plant with a capacity of 150 m^3/day to serve 1500 people was constructed. The cost of treatment was estimated at $0.055 per m^3 of treated water.

Edwards studied the removal of As(III) and As(V) using $FeCl_3$, alum and their preformed oxides.[78] As(V) removals were independent of initial As(V) concentration and coagulant dosage, and solely dependent on pH, with maximum removals occurring at 7.0. As (III) removals were found to be dependent on the initial As(III) concentration and the coagulant dosage and independent of the pH. The author suggested surface adsorption as a dominant mechanism for the removal of arsenic by the performed oxides, while both, adsorption and coprecipitation were responsible for arsenic removal by $FeCl_3$ and alum. Another study conducted by Cheng and others used alum and $FeCl_3$ for the removal of As(V) from water.[135] Bench, pilot and demonstration scale studies were conducted using coagulant dosage of 10, 20 and 30 mg/L at pH values of 7.0, 6.3 and 5.5. Arsenic removal was found to be dependent on pH. coagulant dosage and turbidity of the raw water. As(V) removals were poor for water with high turbidity and was prominent when <20 mg/L coagulant dosages were used. $FeCl_3$ was more effective than alum for the removal of arsenic from water. As (V) removal by alum was found to be pH dependent, with maximum removals observed at pH <7. Removal of As (V) with $FeCl_3$ was not pH dependent and increased with increasing coagulant dosage.

Kanbar studied simultaneous iron and As (III) removals using oxidation, coagulation, settling, filtration, and membrane filtration.[129] Tap water was spiked to As(III) concentration of 0.2 mg/L and Fe(II) concentration of 1 mg/L. The order of effectiveness of oxidants for the simultaneous removal of As (III) and iron was found to be: $KMnO_4 > O_3 > NaOCl > O_2$. The most effective inorganic coagulants for arsenic removal were found to be $CuSO_4$, $CuCl_2$, $ZnCl_2$, $FeSO_4$, and $Fe_2(SO_4)_3$. Removals of As(III) were reported to be in the range 75 to 88 per cent after oxidation with $KMnO_4$, NaOCl, or O_3 followed by coagulation, settling and membrane filtration. A cost estimate incorporating oxidation, coagulation and filtration indicated an operational cost of $0.33 per 100 gallon and a capital and operational cost of $0.46 per 1000 gal. treated.

Chang and others concluded that ferric chloride was more effective than alum for the removal of arsenic from groundwater.[124] A 15-minute flocculation test performed using shallow aquifer groundwater with a total organic carbon (TOC) of 0.5 mg/L, spiked to 50 µg/L arsenic, indicated no settleable floc formation for ferric chloride and alum dosages below 40 mg/L and 80 mg/L respectively. This phenomenon was attributed to the low particulate content of the groundwater. Blended groundwater with a TOC of 3.5 mg/L was found to impair arsenic removal for coagulant dosages less than 20 mg/L; higher TOC however enhanced arsenic removals for coagulant dosages above 40 mg/L.

Coagulation was studied for the removal of arsenic from waters containing 50 mg/L arsenic.[130, 131] Coagulation and precipitation experiments were performed using silver, copper, magnesium, aluminum and iron salts. Results indicated over 80 per cent removal for As(III) using copper and silver salts. Copper salts ($CuSO_4.5H_2O$), however, gave higher removals of arsenic than silver salts (Ag_2SO_4). Neutral pH values gave maximum arsenic removals.

Though coagulation is a popular method for arsenic removal, it suffers from problems of sludge disposal and cannot be readily applied to small and intermittent flows.

10.2 Lime Softening

Table 6 presents a summary of arsenic removal by lime treatment.

Table 6: Arsenic Removal by Lime Treatment

Arsenic Species	Treatment Method	Initial Conc. (mg/L)	Removal (Per cent)	pH	Reference
As(V)	Excess lime softening	12	95	10.6–11.4	121
As (V)	Lime	0.4	40–70	9.0–10.0	121
As (V)	Lime	5	80	10.0	136
As (V)	Lime	5	76	11.5	136

Logsdon and Symons studied removal of As (V) from water using lime and excess lime softening.[121] River water, well water and tap water samples were spiked to achieve As (V) concentration from 0.1 to 20 mg/L. As (V) removals of 40–70 per cent were reported by lime softening in the pH range of 9 to 10. Removals, however, increased when lime softening was followed by iron coagulation. Excess lime softening showed the highest As (V) removals in the pH range from 10.6 to 11.4; 95 per cent removals could be achieved for an As(V) concentration of 12 mg/L. Maruyama and others found iron precipitation was more effective than low lime and high lime treatment for the removal of As (III) from domestic wastewater.

Dutta and Chaudhuri reported the use of lime softening with powdered coal additive to lower arsenic concentration (total arsenic 0.68–0.70 mg/L, As(III) 0.59–0.60 mg/L) below the guideline value of 0.05 mg/L.[137] Laboratory tests suggested a lime dosage of 1250 mg/L at pH 11.5 to achieve 90 per cent arsenic removal. On addition of 2 g/L of powdered coal additive and a lime dosage of 800 mg/L (pH 11.5). the residual arsenic concentration was reduced to below 0.05 mg/L. The presence of magnesium assisted in the removal of arsenic and the magnesium hydroxide floc played a significant role in the removal of As(III).

10.3 Activated Alumina (AA) Systems

Activated alumina (AA) has been frequently used for the removal of arsenic from contaminated water supplies. Table 7 presents a summary of arsenic removal by activated alumina treatment.

An activated alumina tank (1 ft³) pilot system was installed in two homes in Eugene, Oregon and the other in Fairbanks, Alaska, for point-of-use treatment, to remove As(V) occurring at the high levels of 0.05–1.16 mg/L.[118, 138] The AA systems showed initial arsenic removals of 30–40 per cent. The poor performance was attributed to poor

pretreatment of the AA i.e. alumina had not been rinsed
with dilute sulfuric acid after initial washing with caustic.
A follow-up study showed that an influent arsenic
concentration of 0.1 mg/L was reduced to below 0.05 mg/
L. However, after 420 days of operation of the AA columns,
the arsenic concentration of the effluent was found to be
higher than the MCL indicating that even pretreatment
could not guarantee long-term performance.

Table 7: Arsenic Removal by Activated Alumina Treatment

Arsenic Species	Initial Conc. (mg/L)	Removal (per cent)	pH	Reference
As (V)	5	>99	6.9	77
As (V)	10	99	6.8	77
As (III)	0.5	89	8.47	77
As (III)	1	83	8.04	77
As (III)	2	79	8.20	77
As (V)	2.4	100	6.8	77
As (V)	0.1–0.4	>90	5.0	75
*	0.05–1.16	30–40	*	118, 138
*	0.1	>50	*	118, 138
*	0.08–0.116	*	5.5	139
*	0.06	95	7.1	140
Dimethyl arsenate	0.75	<70	4.0	141

*: Information or data not given by the authors.

Ginocchio reported the effective use of flocculation/
sedimentation and activated alumina for the removal of
As(V).[75] Over 90 per cent of As(V) was removed by
precipitation using flocculation/sedimentation at pH values
between 6.5 and 7.0 using 5 g/m³ trivalent iron flocculant
admixture. The concentration of As (V) in the raw water

was in the range of 0.1 to 0.4 mg/L. Activated alumina showed highest As(V) removals in the pH range of 5.0 to 5.5. The adsorption capacity of AA for As(V) indicated a specific loading capacity for As(V) of 10–15 mg/dm³. A concentrated caustic soda solution was used for the regeneration of activated alumina.

A pH range from 5.5 to 6.0 was suggested to be the optimum pH range for the removal of arsenic from groundwater by activated alumina.[142] Table 8 presents a summary of As(III) and As(V) removal by activated alumina columns from different groundwater sources. A 40 per cent NaOH solution is recommended for the base regeneration of the spent activated alumina columns and a 2 per cent H_2SO_4 solution for acid neutralization. A regeneration of 50 to 70 per cent has been reported, with the regenerated alumina showing loss in adsorption capacity for arsenic resulting in shorter column runs reducing the breakthrough time by 10–15 per cent.

Table 8: As(III) and As(V) Removal from Groundwater Sources by Activated Alumina[142]

AS(III)	As(V)	Total As	pH	BV Treated to 0.05 mg/L (As)	Total Arsenic Capacity (g/m³)
100	0	100	6.0	300	20
80	10	90	6.0	700	60
31	57	88	6.0	9000	575
0	110	100	5.5	13100	1280
0	98	98	6.0	16000	1410
0	100	100	6.0	23000	1920

Pilot plant studies were conducted at the Fallen, Naval air station (NAS), Nevada, to study the removal of arsenic

(0.08–0.116 mg/L) from the NAS drinking water supply using; granular activated alumina (AA) with pH adjustment to 5.5 and granular activated alumina without pH adjustment.[139] Raw water at a pH of 9.0–9.1 was treated in a downflow, packed bed configuration with an initial flow rate of 1.5 gpm giving an empty bed contact time (EBCT) of 5 min reducing to 1 gpm or 7.5 min. EBCT. The treatment runs were continued until the arsenic level in the treated water was at or near the arsenic level in the raw water. Based on the study, activated alumina treatment with pH adjustment to 5.5 was found to be the best available option. The authors found that a potential existed for blending 50 per cent treated water with 50 per cent raw water, and observed a 75:25 ratio of treated to raw water could be used for a conservative design. Regeneration of the activated alumina columns resulted in a toxic waste containing ≥ 5 mg/L of soluble arsenic. Arsenic was removed by precipitation from this waste in the pH range of 5.0–6.6, resulting in a supernatant arsenic concentration of 0.01 mg/ L. The operation and maintenance costs per 1000 gallon for activated alumina treatment with pH control at 5.5 at flow rates of 700, 2400 and 100 gpm were estimated at $0.221, $0.318 and $0.298 respectively. The capital costs corresponding to the above flow rates were estimated at $558,000, $1,343,000 and $179,000 respectively.

An initial arsenic concentration of 0.06 mg/L was reduced to 0.003 mg/L using activated alumina treatment.[140] Reducing the pH of the influent raw water from 9.3 to 7.1 aided the removal process significantly. It was observed that at higher arsenic levels (0.5 mg/L) arsenic removal decreased initially, occasionally depending on the initial pH to an effluent concentration of 0.01 mg/L and increased thereafter. This phenomenon was attributed to the interruption in flows which resulted in enhanced exchange capacity. Operating costs based on chemical costs alone were estimated at US$15–US$50 per million gallons treated.

Adsorption of As(V), methyl arsenate and dimethyl arsenate by activated alumina was studied.[143] The affinity of the adsorbates to the adsorbents decreased in the following order: As(V) > methyl arsenate > dimethyl arsenate.

Batch kinetic studies using activated alumina indicated that the rate of uptake of As(III) was much slower in comparison to As(V).[77] The initial concentrations of As(III) and As(V) were varied from 0.4 to 10 mg/L. The uptake of As(V) by activated alumina was studied in the pH range of 4.0 to 7.0 and the optimum pH range for the uptake of As(V) was found to be 6.0 to 7.0. Removal of As(III) by activated alumina was studied in the pH range from 4.0 to 9.0; the optimum pH range was found to be 6.5 to 8.5. High removals were observed for As(V) than As(III), and pretreatment by chlorine oxidation of arsenite to arsenate prior to adsorption was suggested.

Cox and Ghosh[141] studied surface complexation of methyl arsenate and dimethyl arsenate by activated alumina. Batch adsorption experiments suggested an equilibrium adsorption time of four hours, when 95 per cent removals were observed. The point of zero charge (PZC) for activated alumina was found to be 8.1. Adsorption of methylated arsenates was found to decrease with increasing pH and initial arsenic concentrations. An initial concentration of 1.0×10^{-5} M dimethyl arsenate showed less than 70 per cent removals with activated alumina. Based on the study, a model was developed to describe adsorption equilibria as a function of pH, ionic strength and adsorbate-adsorbent ratio. They suggested a two site triple-layer model which could be used to describe the adsorption behaviour.

10.4 Adsorption

The potential of activated carbon to remove arsenic from water supplies has been suggested to be very good, depending mainly on the oxidation state of arsenic.[144] Table 9 presents a summary of arsenic removal by adsorption.

Lignite based activated carbon, characterised by high ash content (22.1 per cent on dry basis) effectively removed As(V) from water and removals were about five times as much as those observed using carbons with low ash content (0.15 per cent on dry basis).[145] As the ash content in the carbon increased, the adsorption capacity of the carbon increased reaching a plateau at 10.5 mg As/g carbon. The main mechanism of removal was suggested to be a strong interaction between arsenic and the mineral matter on the carbon ash. A chitin/chitosan mixture was studied as a potential agent for the removal of arsenic from contaminated groundwater in Halifax. Nova Scotia. Canada.[146] Adsorption experiments were conducted using well water at pH 7.5, spiked to As(III) concentrations ranging from 0.1 to 0.3 mg/L. A chitin to chitosan ratio of 1:1 resulted in the reduction of As (III) from 0.1 mg/L to 0.04 mg/L. The capacity of the mixture at pH 7 was found to be 0.13 µg As/g. Greater than 95 per cent of the arsenic in the spent adsorbent and effluent from the treatment column was found to be in the +5 oxidation state. The major mechanism of arsenic removal was suggested to be a combination of ion exchange and chelation. The arsenic removal capacity of the chitin/chitosan mixture was reported to be 10,000 times less than ion exchange resins.

Table 9: Arsenic Removal by Adsorption

Arsenic Species	Treatment Method	Initial Conc. (mg/L)	Removal (Per cent)	pH	Reference
As(V)	Activated carbon	0.96	96.5	3.1	77
As(V)	Activated carbon	1.9	92.4	3.1	77
As(V)	Activated carbon	2.6	83.5	3.2	77
As(III)	Activated bauxite	0.49	79.6	8	77
As(III)	Activated bauxite	1	73	7.7	77
As(III)	Activated bauxite	2	70	7.8	77
As(V)	Activated bauxite	4.5	99	6.7	77
As(V)	Activated bauxite	7.8	97	6.8	77
Dimethyl arsenate	Hydrated ferric oxide	3.7	>95	4.0	141
Methyl arsenate	Hydrated ferric oxide	97	=100	4.0	141
As(V)	Lignite based	7.5	10.5 mg As/g carbon	7.1–7.2	145
As (III)	Chitin/Chitosan mixture	0.1	60	7.5	146
As(V)	Granular activated carbon	7.5	12 to 61	4.0	148
As(V)	Powdered activated carbon	3.7	5 to 84	4.0	148

Adsorption of As(V), methyl arsenate and dimethyl arsenate by kaolinite clay and ferric hydroxide was studied.[143] Ferric hydroxide was found to have the highest adsorption capacity for the organo arsenicals than kaolinite clay. The affinity of the adsorbates to the adsorbents decreased in the following order:

As(V) > methyl arsenate > dimethyl arsenate.

Over 95 per cent removals of 5×10^{-5} M dimethyl arsenate by hydrated ferric oxide was observed at a pH of 4.0.[137] Almost complete removal of 1.3×10^{-3} M methyl arsenate was observed using hydrated ferric oxide at a pH of 4.0. Arsenate removals were found to increase with decreasing initial concentrations.

The rate of uptake by activated bauxite and activated carbon for As(III) was much slower in comparison to As(V).[77] The uptake of As(V) by activated bauxite was found to be a maximum in the pH range from 6.0 to 7.0. The optimum pH range for the uptake of As(V) by activated carbon was found to be 3.0 to 4.0. High removals were observed for As(V) than As(III), and pretreatment by chlorine oxidation of arsenite to arsenate prior to adsorption was suggested. Adsorption of As(III) and As(V) by alumina (Al_2O_3), titanium dioxide (TiO_2) and their mixtures treated chemically with iron hydroxide $[Fe(OH)_3]$, from drinking water has been reported.[147] Batch and column experiments were conducted to determine the effectiveness of the adsorbents. Batch kinetic experiments suggested an equilibrium contact time of 18 h. for the removal of 0.2 mg/L As(III) by pretreated Al_2O_3, TiO_2 or a 80:20 ratio of Al_2CO_3, TiO_2 or As(V) by pretreated TiO_2 at a pH of 7.2 and 25±0.5°C. Isotherm experiments were conducted by varying the initial As(III) and As(V) concentrations from 1 mg/L to 100 mg/L and mixing with 1 mg of the respective adsorbent at pH 7.2 and temperature 25±0.5°C. Results indicated higher removals for As(V) by the adsorbents as compared to As(III), with pretreated alumina showing the highest adsorption capacity. Regeneration of the adsorbents with 1 M NaOH solution resulted in regeneration efficiency ranging from 34–62 per cent. Increasing the concentration of the regenerant did not improve the regeneration efficiency, suggesting chemisorption of arsenic on the adsorbent surface.

Removals from 12 to 61 per cent were achieved using 5 g/L granular activated carbon with an initial As(V) concentration of 1×10^{-4} M at a pH of 4.0 and an equilibrium adsorption time of 24 hours, while, 5 to 84 per cent As(V) removals were achieved using 1 g/L powdered activated carbon with an initial As(V) concentration of 5×10^{-5} M at a pH of 4.0 and an equilibrium adsorption time of 24 hours.[148] Batch adsorption experiments revealed optimum pH ranging from 4 to 5 for the adsorption of As(V) by activated carbon. The major removal mechanisms suggested were electrostatic attraction and the formation of specific surface bonds. Regeneration of the spent activated carbon was achieved using strong acid or base. Ferrous perchlorate was found to be the most effective pretreatment solution to improve the capacity of activated carbon for the removal of As(V).[149] This pretreatment was found to improve arsenic removal capacity and also the regeneration of the spent carbon.

A laboratory study was carried out by Guha and Chaudhuri to screen low-cost materials (bituminous coal, lignite, crushed coconut shell, illite, kaolinite. rice husk, fly ash, charcoal and sand) for arsenic (III) removal from groundwater (water spiked with 1.0 mg/L arsenic).[150] Based on batch sorption screening test, bituminous coal, crushed coconut shell and sand were selected for column tests. Sand medium was selected for best overall performance and it produced an effluent with arsenic levels below 0.05 mg/L for 32 hours; further studies were recommended.

Singh and others studied the removal of As (III) by natural hematite (particle size below 200 μm) and found that the adsorption of As (III) fitted the Langmuir isotherm[151] however the maximum capacity was only about 2.6 μmol/g (or about 0.2 mg/g As (III). This study shows that As (III) is removable to some extent and suitable natural oxides can be applied for adsorption.[72]

In a further study, Prasad showed that the removal of As(V) from aqueous solution was feasible by adsorption onto geological materials such as hematite and feldspar.[152] His study showed that the removal of arsenic followed first-order kinetics and the Langmuir isotherm was applicable to the adsorption process.

10.5 Ion Exchange

Anion exchange is not economically attractive for water with high total dissolved solids (TDS > 500 mg/L) or sulfate (> 25 mg/L).[142] To make ion exchange process effective, As(III) has to be oxidized to As(V) prior to treatment. The advantages of using ion exchange are that pH adjustment is not required and sodium chloride can be used to elute 80–100 per cent of arsenic from the spent column. Removal of As (V) from groundwater with 0.085 mg/L using ion exchange resins, showed its effectiveness for treatment of 4200 BV (bed volumes) at a 5.6 min. EBCT before the arsenic level in the effluent reached 0.05 mg/L.[142] They suggest 2 BV of 1 N NaCl (7.3 Ib NaCl per cubic foot of resin) for the regeneration of the spent resin with a exchange capacity of 1 equiv./L. Removal of As(V) by chloride form strong base anion-exchange resin and regeneration of the spent resin is given below:[142]

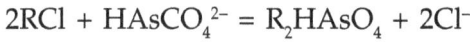

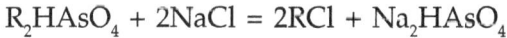

$$2RCl + HAsCO_4^{2-} = R_2HAsO_4 + 2Cl^-$$

$$R_2HAsO_4 + 2NaCl = 2RCl + Na_2HAsO_4$$

Removal and recovery of arsenate and arsenite anions from dilute aqueous solution were studied using a weak base chelating resin (Dow XFS–4195) in ferric ion form by ligand exchange sorption process.[153] The resin, XFS–4195, is a macroporous chelating resin with pendant weak base functional groups used to bind Fe(III) ions. The sorption of As(III) and As (V) was found to be significantly higher by ligand exchange (ion exchange with counterions of Fe(III) followed by complexation with metal ions) than ion exchange. The uptake of As (III) and As (V) by XFS [Fe(III)] was described by the Langmuir and Freundlich isotherms. In a further study on the removal of arsenate and arsenite from aqueous solutions, iminodiacetic chelating resin, Chelex 100 in the ferric form was compared to XFS [Fe(III)].[154] The resin, Chelex 100, has a crosslinked polystyrene macroreticular lattice and a total capacity of 2.9 meq/g dry resin. Adsorption of As (V) and As(III) by Chelex [Fe(III)] was described using Freundlich and Langmuir isotherms. The iron to arsenic ratio for saturation ligand sorption was 1 : 1.2 for As (V) at a pH value of 2 and 1 : 1.9 for As (III) at pH 10. The rate of sorption of As (III) on Chelex [Fe(III)] at mildly alkaline pH was comparable to that on XFS [Fe(III)], while the rate of sorption of As (V) at mildly acidic pH was much higher for XFS [Fe(III)] than Chelex [Fe(III)].

10.6 Reverse Osmosis (RO)

Reverse osmosis (RO) systems comprise a prefilter for sediment removal and if necessary, an activated carbon filter for chlorine removal. These prefilters are followed in turn by a RO membrane, a storage tank and a granular activated carbon system. Table 10 summarises the arsenic removal reported in literature using reverse osmosis treatment.

Table 10: Arsenic Removal by Reverse Osmosis Treatment

Arsenic Species	Treatment Method	Initial Conc. (mg/L)	Removal (Per cent)	pH	Reference
As(III)	Reverse osmosis	0.101	73	*	118
*	Reverse osmosis Reverse osmosis (low pressure, 40–60 psig)	0.5– 1.16	60–80 at startup	*	118, 138
*	Reverse osmosis	0.08	71–93	*	118
*	Reverse osmosis (high pressure, 196 psig)	0.05– 0.016		*	118, 138
As(V)	Reverse osmosis (high pressure, 400 psi)	*	91–98	*	155
As (III)	Reverse osmosis (high pressure, 400 psi)	*	63–70	*	155
As(V)	Reverse osmosis (low pressure, 200 psi)	*	77–87	*	155
As (III)	Reverse osmosis (low pressure, 200 psi)	*	12–35	*	155
As(V)	Nanofiltration at 48 psi and 15 per cent recovery	0.046	> 97	8.5	124
As(V)	Nanofiltration at 49 psi and 30 per cent recovery	0.047	> 97	8.5	124

Contd...

Table 10–Contd...

Arsenic Species	Treatment Method	Initial Conc. (mg/L)	Removal (Per cent)	pH	Reference
As(V)	Reverse osmosis (low pressure, 142 psi, 15 per cent recovery)	0.047	98	8.5	124
As(V)	Reverse osmosis (low pressure, 150 psi, 30 per cent recovery)	0.05	94	8.5	124

Note: (*) not indicated.

Laboratory studies were conducted for the removal of inorganics using an RO system with a 5 µm prefilter to remove suspended material and an activated refilter to remove chlorine.[118, 138] The RO membrane used was a spiral wound polyamide film membrane. Tap water spiked with As(III) to an initial concentration of 0.101 mg/L was pumped at a pressure of 42±2 psi. Arsenic removal of 73.3 per cent was achieved using the system. A field study conducted in the village of San Ysidro, New Mexico for evaluating RO as a point-of-use treatment system, revealed its effective use in arsenic removal, reducing an influent arsenic concentration of 0.068 mg/L to a range below the detectable level (<0.005 mg/L) to 0.02 mg/L.[68] The cost of the RO system employed in the above field projects was $325, with a monthly service contract for $8.60.

Huxstep reported the removal of inorganic contaminants including arsenic from water using high pressure (400 psi) and low pressure (200 psi) reverse osmosis (RO) systems, having a rated capacity of 1.82 L/s of product water.[155] He studied the removal of As (III) and As(V) in spiked groundwater in test runs lasting from 1 to 5 days. The high pressure system, though it required almost twice the energy as the low pressure system, was found to be more effective in the removal of arsenic. High pressure RO systems achieved 91–98 per cent removals for As(V), whereas removals for low pressure systems ranged from 77 to 87 per cent. The high pressure systems indicated 63 to 70 per cent removals for As(III) with removals in the low pressure systems ranging between 12 to 35 per cent. In summary, the results showed that both the high and low pressure RO systems were effective for the removal of As(V), but not satisfactory for removal of the more toxic As(III). Thus, prior to using RO for drinking water treatment, the speciation chemistry of arsenic in the water should be studied. Clifford and others have reported removal of As(III) and As(V) using various types of RO membranes.[123] They have recommended the oxidation of As (III) to As(V) prior to the use of the process. Removal of As(III) by the various types of membranes varied widely with rejections ranging from 46 to 75 per cent for initial As (III) concentrations in the range from 0.04 to 1.3 mg/L. High rejections (98–99 per cent) were observed using the same membranes for As(V) at initial concentration ranging from 0.11 to 1.9 mg/L. Chang *et al.* found microfiltration to be more effected than conventional filtration for arsenic removal.[124] Nanofiltration membranes were found to be effective for arsenic removal at low (15-30 per cent) recovery levels. They suggested the use of low pressure reverse osmosis membrane for high arsenic removals at high recovery levels. A summary of their results is shown in Table 10.

10.7 Filtration

Table 11 represents a summary of arsenic removal by oxidation and filtration. An AWWA committee report quoted the use of manganese greensand filters for the removal of arsenic along with iron [Fe(II)) in Sudbury, Ontario.[68]

Table 11: Arsenic Removal by Oxidation and Filtration

Arsenic Species	Treatment Method	Initial Conc. (mg/L)	Removal (Per cent)	pH	Reference
*	KMnO$_4$ oxidation 7 hour filtration	0.29	78	7.3	132
*	KMnO$_4$ oxidation 15 hour filtration	0.21	78	7.3	132
*	Chlorine (4.5 mg/L) oxidation and filtration	0.26	> 98	7	132
*	KMnO$_4$ oxidation and manganese greensand filtration (170,000 L)	52	96	7.3	156
As (III)	KMnO$_4$ (1 mg/L) oxidation, 2 hour manganese greensand filtration	0.11	91	7.2	157
As (III)	KMnO$_4$ (1.5 mg/L) oxidation, 2 hour manganese greensand filtration	0.135	92	7.2	157
As(III)	KMnO$_4$ oxidation and manganese greensand filtration (400 bed volumes), Fe: As-20 : 1	0.2	> 97.5	*	158
As (III)	KMnO$_4$ oxidation and manganese greensand filtration (400 bed volumes), Fe: As-20 : 1	0.025	>80	*	158
As (III)	KMnO$_4$ oxidation and manganese greensand filtration (400 bed volumes), Fe: As-0 : 1	0.025	45.2	*	158

Note: *: Information or data not given by the authors.

The report acknowledged the need to find a suitable treatment method for the removal of arsenic from water in small communities. Contact adsorption concentration of oxidized iron, manganese and As(V) from 2.40 mg/L. 0.10 mg/L and 0.210 mg/L to 0.06 mg/L, 0.03 mg/L, and 0.01 mg/L respectively, at a pH of 7.3.[132] Chlorine and potassium permanganate were used to oxidize Fe(II) to Fe(III), Mn(II) to Mn(IV) and As(III) to As(V). The flow rates applied to the clarifier and filter were 10 gpm/ft^2 and 5 gpm/ft^2 respectively. An iron to arsenic ratio of 10:1 resulted in the reduction of 0.26 mg/L of arsenic to less than 0.005 mg/L at a pH of 7.0. When potassium permanganate was used, the oxide coated adsorption clarifier and filter media promoted "greensand" effect. Arsenic removal was found to be dependent on the iron to arsenic ratio. A higher iron to arsenic ratio improved arsenic removals.

Laboratory studies confirmed high arsenic removals using KMnO$_4$ oxidation followed by manganese greensand filtration.[157] Physical-chemical adsorption of arsenic to the iron and manganese oxide was suggested to be the main mechanism for the removal. The adsorption of arsenic to manganese oxide may be a dominant mechanism in the removal process. Limited studies on the effect of iron concentration on arsenic removal did not give conclusive results.

Continuous and intermittent regeneration of greensand filters with potassium permanganate was effective for the removal of As(III) at varying initial concentrations.[158] The continuous regeneration process allows for the oxidation of As(III) to As (V) prior to reaching the filter, while the intermittent regeneration process depends on the media bed for the oxidation and finally adsorption of As (V). Presence of iron was found to enhance the arsenic removal process. An initial As(III) concentration of 200 µg/L was reduced effectively below a detection limit of 5 µg/L for over 400 bed volumes using intermittently regenerated greensand. The initial iron and manganese concentration in the feed was 4 mg/L each. The iron to arsenic ratio in this study was 20:1. As the iron to arsenic ratio decreased to 10:1 the arsenic removed in over 400 bed volume was 90 per cent (20 µg/L in effluent). An iron to arsenic ratio of 25:1 was recommended for the removal of arsenic using greensand filters. An initial As (III) concentration of 25 µg/L was reduced below a detection limit of 5 µg/L by greensand filtration using an iron to arsenic ratio of >20:1 for over 400 bed volumes at flow rates of 3 gpm/ft² and 7 gpm/ft². The length of filter runs depended on the flow rates while arsenic removal efficiencies were independent of the flow rates. Potassium permanganate dosages used and the pH of the influent water have not been mentioned. To confirm the effect of iron on arsenic removal, a filter run was carried out with no iron or manganese in the raw water containing 25 µg/L of arsenic. Arsenic removal of 45.2 per cent was observed in this run. Based on the outcome of these results, a pilot scale study was conducted at a water treatment plant. The water to be treated had 0.8 mg/L iron, 0.04 mg/L manganese and 30 µg/L arsenic. The study indicated an effective use of the treatment method lowering the arsenic concentration to 8 µg/L and iron to 0.02 mg/L. The manganese level in the treated water remained at 0.04 mg/L which was attributed to the overfeed of potassium permanganate.

A pilot study at a well site in the village of Harvey, New Brunswick, Canada used chlorine oxidation, iron and alum coagulation to react with arsenic in groundwater, making it insoluble and subsequently removing by filtration using a unique media having a high affinity for metallic ions.[159] The process was found to be effective for the removal of arsenic, lowering an initial arsenic concentration of 61 µg/L to 15 µg/L. The optimum chemical dosages for the removal of arsenic was 6 mg/L chlorine, 2.5 mg/L iron, 2 mg/L alum and filtration at 5 USgpm/ft². An iron to arsenic ratio of 30:1 was suggested for high arsenic removals. The filtration media was also effective for the removal of iron and manganese. On treatment, an increase in hardness was found and no explanation was given for this behaviour. A summary of the results is shown in Table 12.

Table 12: Summary of Removal of Various Contaminants Using Chlorine Oxidation, Iron and Alum Coagulation and Filtration Using a Unique Media from Groundwater[159]

Parameter	Influent Conc. (mg/L)	Effluent Conc. (mg/L)
Hardness	133	156
Total organic carbon	1	0.9
Sulfate	9	9
Chloride	50.3	48.2
Arsenic	0.061	0.015
Iron	2.46	0.03
Manganese	0.01	<0.01
Copper	0.02	0.01
Zinc	0.10	0.01

A recent study showed that arsenic III was easily oxidized by manganese oxides and that the oxidation of

As(III) followed a second order rate law.[160] Flow through tests in small sand filters loaded with manganese dioxide showed a decreasing oxidation of As (III) in the first 60 hours, followed by an increase in oxidation, possibly caused by bacterial action; the release of soluble manganese in the effluent was found to be low.

10.8　Summary of Arsenic Removal Technologies

In general, removal of As (III) is lower as compared to the removal of As(V). Being a nonionic species in the neutral pH zone As(III) is not removed by adsorption since no electrostatic attraction exists and the number of adsorption sites available for As(III) are less than that for As(V).[161] This makes it important to identify the species of arsenic before selecting the treatment scheme. The valence state of arsenic is very important in determining the optimum treatment process to be incorporated, since the arsenic removal efficiency of most of the conventional processes are valence dependent. Oxidation of As(III) using chlorine, potassium permanganate, ozone and other oxidants to As (V) and removal by any of the treatment options available is generally followed. As mentioned earlier, methylated or organic arsenic occurs at concentrations less than 1 µg/L and is not of major significance in drinking water treatment. So far, only limited work has been done to identify the specific forms of arsenic found in drinking water supplies.

Coagulation and lime softening have been studied extensively for the removal of arsenic. Adsorption-coprecipitation with hydrolyzing metals such as Al^{3+} and Fe^{3+} is the most commonly used treatment technique for removing arsenic from water. Iron coagulation achieves higher As(III) and As(V) removal than alum coagulation.

Studies on the use of treatment processes such as reverse osmosis, ion exchange, adsorption or electrodialysis are limited. Available data indicates that high pressure RO systems are more effective compared to low pressure RO systems. Since arsenic occurs as an anion, it can only be removed by anion exchange resins. Neither the household water softeners nor the conventional zeolite softener systems can remove arsenic from water. Ion exchange for the removal of arsenic results in the retention of other anions in the water supply and loses its capacity for arsenic eventually. Activated carbon adsorption is not effective for the removal of arsenic, but pretreatment of activated carbon with iron salts has been shown to improve the sorption capacity for arsenic.

Clifford has summarized (Table 13) the potential for As(III) and As(V) removal using packed beds of activated alumina and strong base resins, reverse osmosis and electrodialysis undermost common pH conditions occurring in groundwater systems.[162]

Table 13: Summary of Methods of Arsenic Removal[162]

Treatment Type	Material	Removals		
		pH	As(III)	As(V)
Packed beds	Activated alumina	5.5–7.5	F–P	G
	Strong base resin	5–9	P	P–G
*Reverse osmosis	Cellulose acetate/ aromatic polyamide membranes	6–8	40–80%	> 80%
*Electrodialysis	–	6–8	40–80%	> 80%

Note : * Removals based on 50–80 per cent recovery;
    G: Good; F: Fair; P: Poor.

The effectiveness of various treatment processes for arsenic removal from water has been summarized by various authors.[163-165] Hamann and others have summarised (Table 14) the general effectiveness of the various water treatment methods.

Table 14: Effectiveness of Water Treatment Processes for Removal of As(III) and As(V)[168]

Treatment Method	As(III)	As(V)
Aeration and stripping	P	P
Coagulation, sedimentation, filtration	F–G	G–E
Lime softening	F–G	G–E
Ion exchange		
Anion	G–E	G–E
Cation	P	P
Membrane processes		
Reverse osmosis	F–G	G–E
Electrodialysis	F–G	G–E
Chemical oxidation and disinfection	P	P
Adsorption		
GAC	F–G	F–G
PAC	P–F	P–F
Activated alumina	G–E	E

E: Excellent; G: Good; F: Fair; P: Poor.

Willey has summarised (Table 15) the treatment technologies available for As(V) and As(III) and their relative treatment costs (based on the construction of new treatment facilities) for 0.3, 1.0, and 50 mgd capacity plants.[166] As can be seen from this Table, ion exchange is the most economical treatment option for smaller capacity treatment plants for removal of As(V), but a trade-off exists in terms of process efficiency (<90 per cent). Alum and iron coagulation are the most cost effective treatment methods for the removal of As (V) in the case of medium to higher capacity plants. Activated alumina treatment is the most efficient amongst the various treatment options resulting in over 95 per cent removals, and could be adapted for smaller capacity plants. However, the regeneration of the adsorbent results in loss of its adsorption capacity. Also, considerable loss of alumina during regeneration occurs due to the formation of sodium aluminate.[125]

Table 15: Treatment Technologies for the Removal of Arsenic and their Relative Treatment Costs[166]

Arsenic Species	Treatment Method	Percentage Removal	Relative Treatment Cost, (Cents/ 1000 gallons)		
			0.3 mgd	1.0 mgd	50 mgd
As (V) (Arsenate)	Alum coagulation/ filtration, pH 6–7	>90	175	44	19
	Iron coagulation/ filtration, pH 6–8	>90	175	44	19
	Excess lime softening	>90	305	63	40
	Activated alumina, pH 5–6	>95	122	62	51
	Ion exchange	<90	83	51	42
	Reverse osmosis	<90	332	164	129

Note: For As(III), oxidation treatment of As(III) to As(V) and use same treatment list for As(V).

The occurrence of As (III) and As(V) of geologic origin in the raw water supply, especially in groundwater, is a major problem in certain regions of Asia such as West

Bengal, India[38,39] and Xinj iang, China[58] and economical removal of arsenic from drinking water using simple and appropriate technologies offers one of the best solutions; other option, of course, is to search for a water source without arsenic. Anthropogenic arsenic pollution by industrial wastes as indicated in the groundwater survey in Chennai, India[40] may not be such a serious problem in the region at present, but may become one if proper measures are not followed to prevent groundwater contamination from industrial effluents.

Conventional water treatment plants (generally used in large communities) employing coagulation, sedimentation and filtration will be usually effective in arsenic removal. The problem becomes serious in small communities in developing countries of Asia and other parts of the world, where wastewater treatment systems for groundwater are either non-existent or simple with only disinfection. In these circumstances, simple treatment systems using filtration techniques with local media such as natural oxides (hematite, manganese and iron oxides) may be the best option.[150, 167, 152, 151] In this context, manganese greensand media may be appropriate in many cases.

Simplicity and cost are the two major factors that should influence the selection of a treatment system for arsenic removal in rural communities dependent on groundwater. Although ion-exchange system may be economical based on an analysis conducted in the U.S.A. such systems may not be appropriate for rural areas in developing countries at this time.

Many treatment schemes can be effective for the removal of a specific inorganic contaminants but no single treatment technique has been found to be effective for all of them. Pilot tests should be conducted prior to selection of a specific treatment process. Rural communities depend on groundwater as a drinking water source and arsenic occurs along with iron and manganese. Oxidation followed by manganese greensand filtration is a very common treatment method for these communities for the removal of iron and manganese. Laboratory, pilot scale, and field studies have shown that arsenic can be removed effectively by these systems to acceptable levels.

10.9 Some Important Observations on Arsenic Removal Technologies

The literature survey reveals that most of the work on arsenic removal has been carried out under laboratory conditions using synthetic waters. These studies show that the efficiency of arsenic removal in different treatment technologies is dependent on the valence form in which arsenic is present in the raw water. Arsenic is present in natural waters either in the inorganic form as arsenate or arsenite, or in the organic form as monomethyiarsenic acid (MMA) and dimethylarsenic acid (DMA). It is evident from the conflicting results reported in the literature that the determination of trace levels of As(III), As (V), MMA and DMA in environmental samples is a difficult analytical exercise and subject to a number of interferences. A recommended method for the determination of arsenic species is described under Annexure II. The studies carried out by Mandal *et al.*[117] in West Bengal has shown that arsenic is present only in the inorganic form (as arsenite and arsenate) and that the organic form of arsenic is absent in the groundwaters in the areas surveyed by them.

Literature further reveals that it is the process of coagulation by ferric salts which has been mainly used in the field studies and in different water treatment plants for the removal of arsenic from drinking waters. The arsenic removal plant installed at Sujapur in the Malda district of West Bengal is also based on the same principle. The raw water here is subjected to pre-chlorination in order to oxidise the As(III) to As(V) because arsenic removal is better for As(V). This is followed by precipitation of As(V) by ferric chloride. The details of arsenic removal plant at Sujapur are described under Section 12.1.

The US-EPA report[120] published in 1978 has summarised that coagulation with iron and aluminium salts, and lime softening are the most effective treatment processes for removing arsenic from water to meet the earlier permissible limit of 50 µg/L of arsenic. However, to ascertain whether these treatment processes can bring down the arsenic level to the present permissible limit of arsenic (10 µg/L) in drinking water requires to be confirmed by further studies. In case these treatment processes are not capable of bringing down the arsenic level to 10 µg/L then a secondary polishing treatment such as ion exchange or activated alumina adsorption may have to be adopted. However, this requires further R&D efforts to be focussed in this direction.

10.10 Limitations of Existing Remediation Technologies

It needs to be emphasized that only a few de-arsenification technologies in vogue have been successfully demonstrated in the field. Most of the existing technologies have severe limitations including high cost, sludge disposal, chemical handling requirements, waste brine disposal, water rejection in water scarce region, etc. Keeping in view these limitations associated with various technologies like coagulation, adsorption using activated alumina, ion exchange, reverse osmosis, nanofiltration and electro dialysis, it becomes imperative to develop efficient de-arsenification technologies based on new processes or advanced functionalized materials.

In this connection, it needs to be reiterated that global interest in improved methods of arsenic removal has led to a rich period of experimentation, in which novel sorbents have been assayed, and existing technologies for arsenic removal modified and/or combined to yield substantially different systems. These novel systems have typically been evaluated only by a handful of researchers, under a narrow range of environmental conditions, for short periods of time. In many cases, advances in removal of arsenic, particularly of arsenite, has been demonstrated, but mechanism are still poorly understood. Much more research needs to be conducted to identify these technologies that can effectively remove arsenic under real-world conditions, and consistently do so for extended periods of time. The biggest challenges ahead lie with development of :

   ☆ Robust affordable household filters for arsenic removal at domestic levels.

   ☆ Feasible treatment technologies for removal of arsenic from wells at community level.

   ☆ Cost-effective and efficient point-of-use and point-of-entry treatment units for arsenic.

The newly developed de-arsenification technologies should be able to provide safe drinking water to poor, rural settings at community levels.

10.11 Future Challenges

Arsenic crisis is a global problem and the solution is in development of breakthrough technologies. In this connection, two major areas contributing significantly towards de-arsenification includes molecularly engineered materials and biotechnological advancements. Self-assembled monolayers on mesoporous materials (SAMMS) is an award winning technology developed by PNNL, USA for removal of arsenic from water with fast kinetics (0.1 s), enhanced adsorption and excellent selectivity which needs to be further tested for their field applications. Another field of interest is the use of genetic engineering to create plants that could clean arsenic from contaminated soils and groundwater. By inserting two bacterial genes into thale cress, Arabidopsis thailana, US researchers have created a plant that not only grows well in the presence of arsenic but also is able to store the toxin in its leaves. [258]

An enzyme directly responsible for converting arsenite to arsenate has been recently discovered. Efforts are underway to identify the same enzyme in other microbes. Also other proteins and genes involved in consuming arsenate are being explored. These findings are to be used to set up bioremediation system for cleaning up mining waste water and also provide safer drinking water for areas such as Bangladesh and West Bengal.

Chapter 11
Safe Disposal of Arsenic–Bearing Sludge

Sludge generated from the treatment of arsenic contaminated groundwater has significant amount of arsenic and requires further treatment before disposal. Solidification and stabilization with cementatious materials is a widely accepted and economically attractive option for disposal of wastes containing heavy metals. Solidification and stabilization (S/S) technique is used to transform hazardous waste into less hazardous or non-hazardous solids for disposal in a landfill. Compressive strength and leach tests need to be conducted on solidified/stabilized test cubes to evaluate the efficiency of treatment techniques. In general solidification technique eliminates free liquid, increases the bearing strength, decreases the surface area of the waste material and produces a monolithic solid product of high structural integrity, whereas stabilization process reduces hazard, potential of the waste by converting the contaminants into their least soluble, immobile and non-toxic form. Other characteristics of the waste would not change by this treatment[259].

Unconfined Compressive Strength (UCS) Test results provide useful information on the ability of the stabilized waste to withstand overburden loads, optimum waste / sludge ratios, curing times for cement setting reactions and improvement in strength characteristics after stabilization of the waste. For chemical fixation of inorganic contaminants especially for anions, the salts in the waste are chemically stable in a wide range of environments. Under field conditions, leaching of hazardous constituents from stabilized/solidified wastes is a function of intrinsic properties of the waste as also the hydrologic and geochemical properties of the site. Laboratory tests are conducted under controlled environmental conditions and hence the leach test results are not directly applicable to leaching behaviour of the wastes in the field. At best, the laboratory leaching data can simulate the behaviour of waste forms under "ideal or static" field conditions. Nevertheless, the results of several leaching tests or of leaching tests combined with physical tests can be used as indicators of field performance and to design waste facilities that will minimize the leaching of hazardous constituents from the waste.

Basu *et al.*[260] studied the leaching potential of two industrial sludges originating from a chemical process plant containing organic polymeric compounds, effluent from an electronic microchip fabrication plant, evaluated the effects of variation of pH and agitation period in the Toxicity Characteristic Leaching Procedure (TCLP). Test on the sludge prior to landfills and concluded that, in general, the amount of release of a particular metal largely depends upon the presence of the metal in the sludge and the standard procedure like TCLP in its present form, does not provide enough information on the leaching potential of the hazardous nature of the sludge in particular landfill.

Trepanowski *et al.*[261] investigated the stabilization of arsenic-bearing soils and wastes using cement casting was effective treatment technology for stabilization of arsenic-bearing sludge. Clay pelletization and sintering technologies are partially successful in stabilizing the arsenic-bearing sludges. Akhter *et al.*[262] studied the leaching of arsenic, cadmium, chromium and lead from solidified/stabilized (S/S) wastes and concluded that Type I ordinary portland cement (OPC) is versatile and dependable agent compared to the other agents viz. fly ash, blast furnace slag and lime. Slag is superior to fly ash in many combinations tested. Interactions with cement in solidification/stabilization of organic and inorganic wastes have been reviewed by Trussell *et al.*[263]. He stated that, solidification/stabilization of inorganic wastes has shown less problem when compared to organic wastes.

Twidwell *et al.*[264] investigated techniques for the treatment of arsenic-bearing solutions and metallurgical solid waste materials at Montana college of Mineral Science and Technology and summarized the studies related to arsenic removal from solutions, stabilization of arsenic bearing waste materials and recovery of arsenic from metallurgical waste and by-products. Andres *et al.*[265] studied the long-term behaviour of stabilized steel foundry dust (SFD) waste which was classified as hazardous and contained lead, chromium, cadmium and zinc. Dynamic Leach Tests (DLT) were performed on solidified/stabilized matrices where portland cement together with anhydrite were used as binders and it was concluded that the mobility of lead was greater than the mobility of zinc.

Dutre *et al.*[266] investigated the leaching mechanism of arsenic from S/S waste by performing static and semi-dynamic leach tests. Calcium plays an important role in the reduction of the leachate concentration through formation of the compound $CaHAsO_3$ in the leachates of the solidified waste material. In the static leach test, the maximum arsenic concentration leached was approximately 25 mg/L and 170 mg/L in the first, second and third leach tests. In the semi-dynamic leach tests, arsenic concentration in the leach for the first leaching period was higher than that for the following periods of leaching. Dutre *et al.*[267] studied the S/S of an industrial waste originating from a metallurgical process in which copper was refined and contained large amounts of arsenic (42 per cent wt). The influence of additives such as waste acid, blast furnace slag, slaked lime, cement, aluminum and barium salts has been studied. The addition of waste acid, slags and the amount of water added had negligible influence on leaching of arsenic from S/S wastes but the addition of lime lowered the leachate concentration in the S/S wastes at various pH ranges. It was found that addition of calcium, alumina and barium salts reduced the leachability of arsenic from the solidified waste and the addition of lime or lime and cement gave the best results.

Buchler *et al.*[268] studied the effect of arsenic compounds on cement hydration reactions and leachability of arsenic in the matrix and reported that organoarsenic compound and arsenic acid had least effect on the formation of the hydrate cement matrix, whereas arsenate and arsenite salts have intermediate effects on matrix formation and low leachability. Akhter *et al.*[269] studied the long term curing time on solidification/stabilization (S/S) of arsenic salts and observed no appreciable change in leachability of arsenic after 3 years of curing, compared with 28 days of curing. Recently studies were undertaken by NEERI at the Zuari Industries Ltd., Goa which included characterization of wastes, assessment of waste disposal site, laboratory-scale treatment and disposal studies, pilot-scale studies, and full-scale treatment and disposal of wastes. The characterization of wastes revealed the presence of very high concentration of arsenic (89000 mg/L). Based on a detailed state-of-the art review, solidification/stabilization was selected as the most techno-economically feasible treatment and disposal option.[270]

Chapter 12
R&D on Arsenic: Indian Scenario

There are several organisations in the country which are engaged in different R&D projects related to arsenic. The details of these projects are presented in Table 16.

As the coordinating laboratory, identified by CSIR, to prepare the base paper on "Control of Arsenic Contamination in Drinking Water", a request letter was issued by NEERI in the year 1997 to all the principal investigators mentioned in the aforementioned Table to highlight the progress/achievements made under their projects. NEERI could get response from only four organisations *viz.*, NML. Jamshedpur, Kalyani University, the Center for Study of Man and Environment (CSME), Kolkata, and the School Of Environmental Studies (SOES), Jadavpur University, Kolkata which has carried out

Table 16: R&D Projects on Arsenic in India (Year 1997)

Sl.No.	Project Title	Name and Address of Principal Investigator
1.	Development alternative sources of potable water in the arsenic affected areas in West Bengal	Dr. Balram Bose Jadavpur University, Mechanical Engg. Deptt. Kolkata – 700 032, West Bengal
2.	Feasibility of utilizing the subsurface water from shallow aquifer in the Gangetic Plains of Uttar Bihar and West Bengal for rural water supply	Prof. K.J. Nath All India Institute of Hygiene and Public Health 110 Chittaranjan Avenue, Calcutta – 700 073, West Bengal
3.	Mechanism of mobilization of arsenic in sedimentary aquifers in West Bengal and realistic approaches for *in situ* remediation methods	Kungi Tekniska Hogs Kolan, Royal Inst. of Technology, Kalyani University, Kalyani, West Bengal
4.	Epidemiological study of chronic toxicity due to arsenic contaminated water in 24 Parganas (South), one of the six arsenic affected districts of West Bengal	Prof. D.N. Guha Mazumdar, Institute of Post Graduate Medical Education and Res. (IPGMER), 244, Acharya J.C. Bose Road, Kolkata – 700 020, West Bengal
5.	Development of low cost filtering medium for the removal of arsenic from groundwater	Sh. S. Bhattacharjee, National Metallurgical Laboratory, Jamshedpur – 831 007, Bihar
6.	Ecology and geochemistry of arsenic occurrences in groundwater of six distt. of West Bengal	A.K. Saha Centre for Study of Man and Environment (CSME), Lake City, Kolkata – 700 091, West Bengal

Contd...

Table 16—Contd...

Sl.No.	Project Title	Name and Address of Principal Investigator
7.	Bio transformation and sink of arsenic from groundwater by microalgal based treatment systems	Dr. Dipankar Chakraborti School of Environmental Studies, Jadavpur University, Kolkata – 700 032, West Bengal
8.	Arsenic in groundwater in six districts of West Bengal	Dr. Dipankar Chakraborti School of Environmental Studies, Jadavpur University, Kolkata – 700 032, West Bengal
9.	Control of arsenic and other chemical pollutants of drinking water	Dr. P.S. Chakraborty, Presidency College, Department of Chemistry, 86/1, College Street Kolkata – 700 073, West Bengal
10.	Arsenic problem in Karnataka	Major Ramesh Public Health Engineering Department (PHED), Anandarao Circle, Bangalore – 660 009, Karnataka

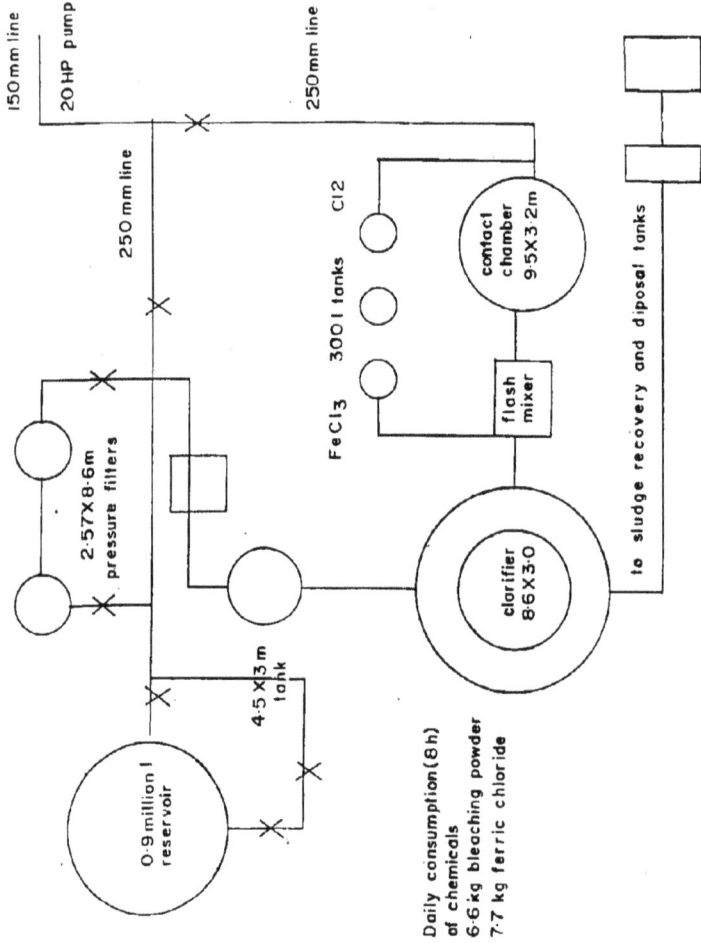

Figure 4: Arsenic Removal Plant at Sujapur, W.B. Government

150 mm line
20 HP pump
250 mm line
250 mm line
Cl_2
$FeCl_3$ 300 l tanks
contact chamber 9·5×3·2m
2·57×8·6m pressure filters
flash mixer
clarifier 8·6×3·0
to sludge recovery and diposal tanks
4·5 ×l3 m tank
0·9 million l reservoir
Daily consumption(8 h)
of chemicals
6·6 kg bleaching powder
7·7 kg ferric chloride

considerable work on arsenic under a CSIR funded scheme. The progress report as submitted by these four organisations on their R&D work related to arsenic is at Annexure III.

Literature review show that significant amount of work has been carried out on arsenic removal in the laboratory as well as in the field by the All India Institute of Hygiene and Public Health (AIIHPH), Kolkata and Environmental Engineering Laboratory, Civil Engineering Department, Bengal Engineering College (Deemed University), Howrah. These two organisations presented research papers highlighting their contributions at the National Workshop sponsored by WHO on "Removal of Arsenic from Drinking Water" held during December 19–20, 1997 at AIIHPH, Calcutta. These two papers alongwith the list of research studies on arsenic contamination in drinking water carried out by AIIH&PH, Kolkata are given under Annexure VI.

12.1 Arsenic Removal Plant at Sujapur, West Bengal

The Public Health Engineering Department (PHED) of West Bengal has installed an arsenic removal plant at Sujapur, in the Malda district of West Bengal. The schematic diagram of this plant is shown in Figure 4.

Chapter 13

Contribution of Council of Scientific and Industrial Research (CSIR)

In the backdrop of the widespread public concern that vast sections of people in the state of West Bengal are exposed to the grave threat of slow arsenic poisoning due to consumption of groundwater containing high concentration of arsenic, the CSIR decided to address the problem as a priority area of R&D. The TABs (Technology Advisory Boards) of the physical and chemical sciences group of laboratories of CSIR, after rigorous scientific deliberations over a period of two years (1995–96), formulated a project proposal entitled "Integrated Water Management for Mitigating Arsenic Contamination in Ground Waters of West Bengal".

The R&D proposal aimed at delineation of a curative strategy comprising technological interventions for reducing arsenic level in drinking water to acceptable limits; and in the long term, implementation of a preventive strategy through sustainable land-water management practices with flood control, water demand management, recharge of aquifers using surplus water available during monsoon months and management of wetlands, as its integral components.

The curative approach focussed on the development of appropriate technologies to reduce the arsenic content in groundwater to around 10 µg/L through a combination of coagulation, precipitation, filtration, ion exchange and adsorption processes, and on development of ecofriendly processes for treatment and disposal of sludge generated during de-arsenification of drinking waters. In keeping with the magnitude of the problem, the technology for de-arsenification was envisaged at three levels, viz. individual household level, spot sources (hand pumps) and centralised treatment system with supply through PSPs.

The key elements of the preventive approach comprised (*i*) preparation of a three dimensional picture of aquifer geometry through geophysical studies, and generation of a database for spatial distribution of arsenic in groundwater for understanding its source and leaching mechanism to facilitate designing long-term mitigation measures; (*ii*) artificial recharge with arsenic free surface water for *in-situ* remediation of contaminated aquifers and (*iii*) delineation of strategies for integrated land and water management practices.

The integrated project submitted by CSIR laboratories was taken up with RGNDWM to mobilise the Government of West Bengal for identifying a nodal agency for interaction and follow up action in implementing the project.

A study on the groundwater development in the arsenic-affected alluvial belt of West Bengal has been made by Mallick and Rajagopal of the HRD Group of CSIR, and their findings are at Annexure IV.

NEERI conducted treatability studies on some groundwater samples collected from the arsenic affected areas of West Bengal and developed a flow sheet for removal of arsenic.[273] The findings of this study are at Annexure V. NEERI has also conducted a study of arsenic contamination in the groundwater of Chowki Block of Rajnandgaon District. Under this study more than 800 groundwater samples were analyzed for arsenic and it was established for the first time by NEERI that the Chowki Block in Rajnandgaon District (earlier in Madhya Pradesh) of Chattisgarh is having the problem of arsenic in groundwater. The detailed report of this study has been submitted by NEERI to PHED, Madhya Pradesh.[274]

R&D pertaining to development of novel hybrid nanomaterials (NHNMs) based on molecular sieves for de-arsenification and molecular imprinting agent for arsenic detection is being pursued at NEERI. Efforts have been made to develop the materials as follows:

☆ Surface modified zeolites by surface treatment of zeolites using surfactant and quarternary ammonium compounds to develop anionic characteristics.

☆ Iron treated zeolite by surface treatment of zeolite with iron salts to form iron-hydroxide and metal nanoparticle impregnated material.

☆ Functionalized treated mesoporous materials by treating MCM-41 with arsenic selective ligands like dimercatosuccinic acid and dimercaptopropanol.

It is expected that these new materials would provide efficient arsenic removal processes to attain the stringent stipulated standard of 10 ppb in different countries.

CSIR and SOES, Jadavpur University have a joint patent for domestic filter tablet system for removal of arsenic from ground water. A large number of requests were received for supply of this system from various agencies within the country and abroad.

The Central Glass and Ceramic Research Institute (CGCRI), Kolkata, has been working on potabilization of surface, sub-surface and arsenic contaminated groundwater, using ceramic membrane technology. The problem of groundwater contamination in West Bengal by arsenic as well as iron was addressed to in this context. As a result of continued efforts, the institute has successfully developed a membrane-based technology for removal of arsenic and iron from groundwater. The technique developed by CGCRI, is essentially a hybrid process consisting of two steps: adsorption of arsenic by a colloidal suspended media and subsequent separation of the media by a ceramic micro filtration membrane. The salient features of this technology are complete removal even upto 40 ppm arsenic content in feed water, generation of minimum sludge volume with ease of entrapped sludge disposal system, modular design enabling installation of medium capacity plant required for covering entire pollution of a large village /outgrowths, continuous operation with elimination of manual labour due to power-operated system. An Indian patent has been filed on this process in March 2001.

A pilot plant based on this technology was installed by CGCRI at Akrampur Talikhola, Barasat, West Bengal, in collaboration with Public Health Engineering Directorate (PHED), Government of West Bengal. Field trials were conducted from 7 January to 13 August 2002, using highly contaminated groundwater, containing iron and arsenic in the range of 9-12 ppm, and 0.9-1.2 ppm respectively for optimization of different operating parameters. The filtered water was found to conform to WHO standards (Fe < 0.3 ppm and As < 0.01 ppm). This has been verified by continuous monitoring of the water quality using spectrophotometry and FI-HG-AAS techniques at Public Health Engineering Directorate, Barasat Division and Jadavpur University, respectively. The pilot plant initially consisted of one multi-element membrane module, having a capacity of 60 LPH. Thereafter, another multi-element module of different configuration was also attached to enhance the capacity of the pilot plant. From February 2002 onwards, every day about 500 litres of filtered water was distributed free of cost among the villagers in 5 litre pet jars to test its acceptability.

After successful field trials by scientists of CGCRI, on 14 August 2002, the pilot plant unit was formally handed over by CGCRI to Barasat Akrampur Human Development Organisation (BAHDO), a local NGO and the land-owner where the unit has been installed, for its maintenance and operation. For increasing the production rate, CGCRI has developed modules containing multi-channel membrane elements, which increase the filtration area from 0.5 (in the case of single channel elements) to 1.7 m^2. To expedite the process of disseminating the technology to the people, two MoUs have been signed with local manufacturers for fabrication of the membrane elements and system design and supply of the plants, respectively. Research was undertaken to develop higher capacity (2500 LPD) plants suitable for community applications. Patents have been filed by CGCRI in some countries affected by arsenic problem like Bangladesh, USA, Taiwan (China) etc.

Several background documents have been published by WHO on the work carried out on arsenic in the groundwaters of West Bengal and Bangladesh. These documents are listed at Annexure VII.

Chapter 14
Recommendations for Future Action

Recognising the gravity of the situation resulting from arsenic contamination of drinking water in Bangladesh, the Government of India in October 1996 convened a special high-level interministerial meeting and constituted a National Steering Committee with the Minister of Health as the Chairman. Various international and donor agencies offered assistance. WHO also supported the visit of a special mission to assist the Central Government and the State of West Bengal, in India/in August 1996 and technical support was provided to Bangladesh through WHO consultants in the last week of April 1997.

As it was felt that the two countries facing arsenic contamination of groundwater would benefit from each other's experiences, a regional consultation on "Arsenic in

Drinking Water and Resulting Arsenic Toxicity in India and Bangladesh" was convened at New Delhi, India, during 29 April–1 May 1997. The consultation brought together key scientific and technical persons from Bangladesh and India as well as international experts for extensive discussions on arsenic problems. A 20-Step Action Plan for achieving the objectives of providing immediate relief to the victims and developing long-term measures for effectively addressing this major public health issue was the outcome of the consultation.

14.1 Recommendations for Action

14.1.1 Preamble

Taking cognizance of the following facts:

1. Arsenic in drinking water is a major public health hazard and should be dealt with as an emergency situation;

2. "Affected people" are those who are showing clinical manifestations, and

3. "People at risk" are those who are drinking arsenic contaminated water and do not necessarily show symptoms of arsenic poisoning.

Relief measures should be provided immediately through:

1. The supply of safe drinking water to all those affected and/or at risk because of current exposure, and

2. Treatment of patients suffering from arsenic poisoning.

Simultaneously, actions must also be initiated for developing long-term measures based on the scientific assessment of factors contributing to the arsenic problem and the identification of appropriate options for its control.

The implementation of both immediate and long-term measures should be decentralized as much as possible with the active involvement of people, affected or at risk, and of local community-based organisations.

14.1.2 Objective I–Immediate Relief Measures

Recommendation 1: Identify Patients and/or Populations at Risk

Organise the identification of patients as well as of the surrounding highly-exposed populations.

Arsenic task forces of adequate strength need to be created to rapidly identify patients with arsenic poisoning. The diagnosis of patients will be made by detecting pigmentation, de-pigmentation or keratosis. The goal will be to identify all the patients in one year.

When the patients have been identified, the surrounding wells should be tested in order to ensure safe water for consumers and to prevent exposure to those who, so far, do not have symptoms of disease.

Special effort should be made to identify arsenic exposure in children and in pregnant and lactating mothers.

Recommendation 2: Provide Symptomatic Treatment

The immediate action for providing symptomatic treatment should include taking care of skin problems, and providing vitamins and nutritious diet. Serious problems should be referred to health centres or regional hospitals.

Recommendation 3: Provide Medical Care at Health Centres for Seriously-Affected Patients

Equipment and medicines must be available at the health centres for managing the seriously-affected patients. Support needs to be made available for this purpose from NGOs and international agencies (*e.g.* WHO, UNICEF and the World Bank).

Recommendation 4: Strengthen Diagnostic Facilities at Regional Level

Many cases of arsenic poisoning are easy to diagnose. In more complicated cases, however, laboratory facilities will need to be improved at the regional level by providing such equipment as atomic absorption spectrophotometer so as to determine the arsenic levels in water as well as human tissues. For this, funds need to be made available from international agencies (*e.g.* WHO, UNICEF, UNDP and the World Bank).

Recommendation 5: Provide Safe Drinking Water

Immediate relief on emergency basis should be provided through the supply of safe drinking water (*e.g.* using tankers and/or introducing domestic treatment of water using appropriate methods of arsenic removal). Intensive information, education and communication (IEC) activities should be undertaken prior to introducing these methods and concurrent monitoring of the effectiveness of these measures should be initiated.

In selecting the source of supply, the following order of preference may be followed:

1. Tubewells proven to be safe (use piped supply or tankers for distribution, wherever necessary).

2. Surface waters (*e.g.* ponds, rivers, canals) with appropriate and adequate treatment.

3. Rain-water harvesting and storage, using locally appropriate and hygienic methods for domestic and community supply.

Organize rapid assessment of water supplies based on all available water quality data and on cases of confirmed or suspected arseniasis so as to identify the "hot spots" needing immediate supply of safe water. Sources with arsenic levels above 0.05 mg/L should be clearly identified for priority action (sources with the highest concentration receiving highest priority). All unsafe sources should be marked and alternate sources of safe water arranged for the community. Particular attention should be paid to patients who should be advised to stop using the contaminated water source.

The arsenic-affected districts will require surveys of the existing water supply for ascertaining the levels of arsenic. The surveys should involve the following two steps:

1. Comprehensive site investigations of all community and private sources using appropriate and reliable field kits to find the presence or absence of arsenic. Irrigation sources should also be evaluated for reference and comparative information, and

2. Laboratory analysis of samples from site investigations so as to establish the exact arsenic levels of field-tested sources.

All of the field data should be compiled, and analysed and entered into a national data bank. In addition to water quality data, hydrogeological information should also be compiled in order to identify the arsenic-containing and arsenic-free aquifers. All this information should be entered into the national arsenic data bank.

Recommendation 6: Build Capacity through Training

Some patients may develop serious complications due to arsenic poisoning but the untrained health personnel may not recognize these for many years. Therefore, in areas having arsenic problems, training should be organised for physicians, medical practitioners and other public health staff of both governmental and nongovernmental bodies for rapid case identification and management.

The key persons in each 'affected' and/or 'at risk' district should be identified as the district-level key trainers (DLKTs) and should be so trained. The DLKTs may include medical personnel, district planning officers, executive engineers, hydrogeologists, college teachers, and NGOs, etc. and should, in turn, train grass root workers at local level.

Appropriate and comprehensive training programmes with curricula and course materials should be developed by the recognised national and regional training institutions.

Recommendation 7: Build Awareness through Mass Communication

Intensive awareness-raising activities should be undertaken immediately with regard to the negative health effects of drinking arsenic-contaminated water in order to introduce preventive measures in cooperation with local bodies, NGOs and others.

All avenues for increasing the awareness in this matter should be utilised, including the mass media and communication facilities of government/nongovernmental organisation(s). Specific posters, leaflets and other communication materials should be developed for this purpose.

Recommendation 8: Implement Comprehensive and Integrated Studies

The activities recommended above should be undertaken in an integrated manner combining the medical and water supply interventions at the district level in order to make the entire district population free from arsenic risks. Comprehensive studies should be initiated in one district, each in Bangladesh and India, with the support of UNICEF, UNDP, the World Bank, WHO and other donors in order to demonstrate the effectiveness of implementing these recommendations.

14.1.3 Objective II–Long-Term Measures

Recommendation 9: Strengthen Inter-ministerial Coordination and Cooperation and Establish Expert Groups

In order to strengthen national level interministerial coordination for addressing problems of arsenic contamination of drinking water, a national apex committee should be formed, or if in existence, be modified, as needed, to effectively involve members of the government and public interest groups for jointly assisting in the development of policies and in the implementation of long-term strategies.

Expert groups should be established for identifying and addressing specific technical and social issues, as required.

Recommendation 10: Establish National Database on Arsenic in Dinking Water and Resulting Arsenic Toxicity

Document the extent of the problem by collecting all the requisite information generated by the investigation projects relating to drinking water supply and health problems and evaluate the data.

Based on such an evaluation, strengthen the national database on arsenic in drinking water. Establish a comprehensive management information system (MIS) to facilitate monitoring and better planning and implementation of programmes.

The data generated by the rapid case identification programme should also be stored and analysed centrally at an appropriate national institution having computer facilities and should form an integral part of the national database and MIS.

Recommendation 11: Review Existing Arsenic Removal Technologies and Evaluate their Efficiency

A number of domestic and community water treatment methods have been developed to remove arsenic in drinking water. A review and evaluation of the arsenic removal treatment technologies and their efficiency should be undertaken with WHO support.

Recommendation 12: Prepare Detailed Site-specific Project Proposals

Prepare detailed site-specific project proposals taking into account the techno-economic feasibility, in order to facilitate the mobilisation of resources and donor support. Efforts should also be made to mobilise support from the private sector and NGOs.

Recommendation 13: Identify Training Needs

Undertake situational analysis of training needs at different levels and establish appropriate mechanisms for capacity-building and institutional development. Include the subject of awareness of arsenic problems in the educational curricula of medical and public health schools. Continuous education of medical, engineering and laboratory staff should be ensured.

Recommendation 14: Establish Appropriate Institutional Framework for Water Quality Surveillance

An institutional framework needs to be developed for regular water quality surveillance and control in the rural and peri-urban areas. A community-based approach dealing with the grassroots should form an integral component of the programme.

Recommendation 15: Establish Appropriate Institutional Framework for Disease Surveillance

An institutional framework needs to be developed for regular surveillance and control of diseases arising out of arsenic poisoning.

Monitor the cases, identify the ongoing exposure and integrate the obtained data with the information available from the drinking water quality surveillance programme. A field kit for testing the presence of arsenic in urine needs to be developed. Monitor the participation of affected persons, PHC personnel, local self government personnel, and the urgent task force personnel. The information, education, and communication (IEC) activities should form an integral part of the disease surveillance and control programme in order that the general public and professional organisations are educated on the problem of arsenic in drinking water. Integrate the arsenic-related disease surveillance into other national disease surveillance programmes (*e.g.* National Cancer Surveillance) and activities relating to nutrition and reproductive health.

Recommendation 16: Establish National Reference Laboratories

Establish national reference laboratories for undertaking the review and evaluation of analytical techniques adopted for the determination of arsenic in drinking water. Also ensure that the quality of data is assured.

Recommendation 17: Support Research Projects

The following research projects have been identified for support:

1. Assessment of the clinical manifestations of chronic arseniasis and the influence on them of various factors.

2. Efficacy of drugs and other means of treatment of arseniasis, including vitamins, nutritious diet, chelation agents and antioxidants.

3. Identification, through epidemiological studies, of the dose-response relationships among skin manifestations in order to determine the safe level of arsenic in drinking water.

4. Identification of factors which make populations susceptible to arseniasis, including nutrition.

5. Long-term cohort study of chronic arseniasis patients to ascertain the rates of progression of latent complications, including cancer.

6. Assessment of the efficacy of the recognised indigenous system of medicine and of homoeopathy in treating chronic arseniasis.

7. Assessment of the risk of exposure to arsenic in the environment and the food chain.

8. Epidemiological study of the affected populations to assess the morbidity patterns with special emphasis on the prevalence of arseniasis in children, pregnant women and lactating mothers.

9. Arsenic removal treatment technologies and their efficiency and cost-effectiveness.

Recommendation 18: Assess the Financial Requirements at National, Provincial and Local Levels

The implementation of the recommendations will require financial resources. Therefore, the financial requirements at the national, provincial and local levels will have to. be assessed, keeping in view the broader perspective of a well-coordinated integrated package of health environment and engineering interventions using cost-effective and locally appropriate technologies and solutions.

Recommendation 19: Establish Bilateral Collaboration

Establish bilateral collaboration between Bangladesh and India for the exchange of geological, chemical, hydrogeological, epidemiological and other technical information. Also establish collaborative visits and other activities of mutual interest.

The exchange of ideas, research data and results of arsenic containment activities should be fostered between governmental agencies, university institutions and research establishments of both countries (Bangladesh and India).

Recommendation 20: Establish International Cooperation and Collaboration

In order to support the implementation of recommendations of this regional consultation, international cooperation and collaboration are felt to be essential. It is, therefore, recommended that international agencies such as UNICEF, WHO, UNDP and the World Bank, etc. as well as bilateral programmes aimed at addressing this major public health hazard.

During December 19-20, 1997 a National Workshop was sponsored by WHO on Technology Options for Removal of Arsenic from Drinking Water which was organised by All India Institute of Hygiene and Public Health, Kolkata in collaboration with PHED, West Bengal. The recommendations outlined in this National Workshop are given below:

1. Removal of total arsenic (arsenite and arsenate) from drinking water is technically feasible by adopting various processes. A few processes are economically viable considering the socio-economic condition of the users.

2. For effective removal of arsenic from drinking water, arsenite if present, need to be oxidised by the application of appropriate oxidants.

3. It has been established that various technologies *e.g.* coagulation-flocculation-sedimentation-filtration (co-precipitation), ion exchange, adsorption, osmosis or electrodyalisis can be used for effective removal of arsenic.

4. Following three types of arsenic removal system can be adopted.

   a. Domestic filter unit

   b. Handpump attached unit

   c. Arsenic removal unit attached with large diameter tubewell for piped water supply scheme

5. As presence of arsenic has been found to be associated with the presence of iron in ground water in West Bengal, adsorption of arsenic on oxidised iron salts takes place during prolonged storage of water. Partial removal of arsenic can be achieved if ground water is stored beyond 24 hours and supernatant is drawn from the storage vessel. Usually rate of removal of arsenic is dependent on duration of storage. However, filtration, after prolonged storage will ensure high removal of arsenic. Such simple method does not require any chemical to be added.

6. Chlorine, sodium hypochlorite, bleaching powder, ozone, potassium permanganate, UV irradiation, etc. can be used as oxidising agent during removal of arsenic from drinking water. Use of sunlight need to be explored thoroughly for household application during removal process.

7. In co-precipitation technique both aluminium sulphate and ferric sulphate are effective. Ferric sulphate has a marginal edge over alum, though alum is readily available in village level at a cheaper cost.

8. Activated alumina has been found to be effective in removal of arsenic and the method does not require addition of any other chemical during the removal process. However, time-to-time regeneration of activated alumina column is necessary and frequency of regeneration is dependent on quantity of water filtered, iron and arsenic content in water. Similarly, activated

carbon can also be used as adsorption media for removal of arsenic.

9. Application of resin for removal of arsenic has been found to be very impressive. In this context, iodised resin has been found most effective not only for removal of arsenic but also for efficient removal of bacteria and iron. However, the frequency of regeneration/replacement of resin is dependent on very many interfering substances present in water.

10. In domestic arsenic removal model, co-precipitation, adsorption and ion exchange process can be used. However, co-precipitation is economically feasible. Either candle filter or sand gravel filter can be used in the domestic model. The sand and gravel filter generally treat more water compared to candle filter. Both the filters can be locally manufactured if the villagers or local artisans are properly trained.

11. Co-precipitation (addition of B.P. solution as oxidant and alum as coagulant) and adsorption technique (activated alumina column) have found to be effective for removal of arsenic from ground water in handpump attached ARP. While the co-precipitation technique is more cost-effective the adsorption technique is more user-friendly. It is found that the capital and recurring expenditures of the co-precipitation model of ARP are more affordable and acceptable to the community.

12. In large diameter tubewell attached arsenic removal plant for piped water supply schemes both the above techniques (co-precipitation and

adsorption) can be adopted. However, the adsorption technique will involve a huge capital and recurring expenditure which may not be economically feasible considering high production cost of the finished water.

13. More number of domestic filter models need to be tested and demonstrated in the field level by involving the community. Direct involvement of Panchayat functionaries/NGOs are emphasised to motivate the user-community.

14. Domestic filters may be procured and maintained by the users through direct contribution. However, minimum subsidy need to be considered for the communities living below the poverty level.

15. Operation and maintenance of handpump attached model should be carried out by the community through their direct participation and contributary fund. A village water committee need to be formed wherever such models would be installed, for looking after the operation and maintenance of the same.

16. R&D on sludge disposal should be undertaken in more rational way to set a guideline for long-term application. However, the sludge can be disposed of in manure pits as an immediate short term measure.

17. More Research and Development studies are still required to be developed in a more rational way for development of low cost removal processes of arsenic from ground water.

18. Feasibility of supplying treated water from traditional surface water sources, if available in arsenic affected areas should receive proper attention. The Horizontal Roughing Filter/Slow Sand Filter developed by AIIH&PH could be used for upgrading the water quality of surface water sources as these sources are free from arsenic contamination.

19. Training on construction and operation and maintenance for different models for technical personnel/panchayat functionaries as well as village level caretakers should be undertaken by the appropriate authorities.

20. A consortium with participatory institutes is to be formed for monitoring and evaluation of the performances of different models including social acceptability.

21. It is recommended to construct a few hand pump attached arsenic removal models and to supply a good number of domestic units in selected villages under current WHO assisted programme for further evaluating technical feasibility, economic viability and social acceptability.

Annexures

Annexure I

Sample Preservation for Arsenic Analysis

Various methods for the preservation of samples for the analysis of arsenic speciation have been reported (Table I.1). Aggett and Kriegman,[169] in a review of. the literature, reported that several authors believed that only minimal sample preservation was needed. For example, in groundwater samples, Tallman and Shaikh[170] reported that the oxidation of As (III) to As(V) was relatively slow, with no oxidation occurring after 3 weeks. Elkhatib *et al.*[85] reported no oxidation of As(III) in soil extracts containing 5 to 500 µg/l of As (III). Seyler and Martin[171] reported that 5 µg/l As (III) was not oxidized at 4°C and pH 7 even after 10 days. In contrast, Andreae[89] reported that at 0.05 µg/l loss of As(III) was detectable after about 1 week and that acidification increased the rate of oxidation. Andreae

Table I.I: Comparison of Published Methods for Preservation of As (III) in Water

Method of Preservation	Results	Reference
None	Oxidation of As(III) to As(V) relatively slow with no oxidation occurring after 3 weeks	170
	No oxidation of As(III) in soil extracts containing 5 to 500 µg/l of arsenic	85
	Below 0.05 µg/l As(III),a loss of As (III) becomes detectable after about 1 week and acidification increases the rate of oxidation	89
	At 1–10 mg/ml samples of As(III) oxidized completely within 4 days	172
	As (III) oxidized within 5 h when present at µg/l level in soil pore water	84
	Losses of Fe and As more or less immediate at room temperature	173
4°C and pH 7	No oxidation of As(III) after 10 days	171
−15°C or under dry ice	An initial loss of about 0.02 µg/l As (III), then unchanged with prolonged storage	89
Filtering, acidifying to pH2 and flushing with nitrogen	Adequate for lake water but unable to prevent some oxidation of As(III) in interstitial water recommended as best method	80, 174, 175
Refrigeration or acidification to pH 2 with HCL	Not adequate to preserve sample 80 for more than a few hours	80

recommended storing the samples at –15°C or under dry ice. Feldman[172] reported that unpreserved samples, containing 1 to 10 μg/l of As (III), oxidized completely within 4 days and Haswell *et al.*[144] reported that As (III) was oxidized in 5 h when present at the microgram per liter level in soil pore water.

Aggett and O'Brien[173] preserved samples of lake water and sediment interstitial water by filtering, acidifying to pH 2, and flushing with nitrogen. This procedure was adequate for lake water but was apparently unable to prevent some oxidation of As(III) in interstitial water.[80] These authors demonstrated that, without any preservation, losses of iron and arsenic were more or less immediate at room temperature.

Likewise, refrigeration or acidification to pH 2 with HCL was not adequate per se to preserve the sample for more than a few hours. Aggett and Kriegman[80] concluded that refrigeration (without freezing) to 2°C, acidification to pH 2 with HCL, and exclusion of air from the sample was the best method to ensure that the sample was adequately preserved. This same procedure has also been reported as acceptable by others workers.[174] These data have significant implications for sampling groundwater because, as noted previously, it is expected to behave more like interstitial water rather than lake water.

A recent study examined the photochemical decomposition of As(III).[176] The half-life for conversion of As(III) to As(V) was 5 min in seawater and 2 min in distilled water. These reactions were performed under a mercury lamp, which is deficient in some of the solar wavelengths. Still, the study shows that exposure to sunlight during sample handling may have a role in the variable results that have been reported.

Another explanation for the variable success of sample preservation reported in the various studies is the effect of manganese. Many samples of reducing groundwater are likely to contain manganese, which is capable of oxidizing As(III).[177]

It is evident, therefore, chat preservation of samples for the determination of arsenic species is dependent on a number of factors ranging from the composition of the sample to whether the sample container was exposed to sunlight. These variabilities explain how a preservation technique that was successful for one experiment might fail under different, yet similar, environmental conditions. Clearly, a priori assumptions on the adequacy of sample preservation may result in significant errors.

Annexure II
Methods for Arsenic Analysis

II.1 Methods for Total Arsenic

One early very common method for the determination of total arsenic was the Gutzeit method.[178]

Spectrophotometry using the silver diethyldithiocarbamate (SDDC) complex of arsine is the classical method for determining arsenic in the 1-100 microgram range.[179] Arsenic is reduced to arsine by either granular zinc in hydrochloric acid or by sodium borohydride. Arsine reacts with SDDC in pyridine and the absorption of the red coloured complex is read at 533 nm. Methylarsine and dimethylarsine, but not trimethylarsine, form SDDC complexes which absorbs at 533 nm, but their complexes have lower molar absorptivities.

A large number of studies can be found in the literature concerning the use of the SDDC method as it is often designated a standard method of analysis.[180] Some more recent papers include one in which the somewhat disagreeable pyridine solvent was replaced by L-erythro-2-(methylamine)-1-phenylpropan-1-ol (L-ephedrine) in chloroform.[181, 182, 183, 184] Ionic interference in the SDDC procedure has been studied by Sandhu and Nelson.[184]

The arsenate ion reacts with ammonium molybdate to form a complex which, when reduced, gives a blue colour.[185] Under favourable conditions, the limit of detection is near 0.1 µg. An adaptation of the method has been used to determine the amounts of phosphate, arsenate and arsenite in sea water.[186] The method is applicable to sea water samples with arsenic concentrations below 3×10^{-6} mol/litre. Precision is of the order of $\pm 0.015 \times 10^{-6}$ mot/litre.

Atomic absorption spectrophotometry (AAS) is a popular method for the determination of total arsenic. Sensitivity of the ordinary flame type AAS for arsenic in solution is comparatively poor, detection limits are in the 0.5–1 mg/litre range.[187, 188] When an electrodeless discharge lamp and an argon-air-hydrogen flame are used, the detection limit is reduced to 0.1 mg/litre.[189] With a long-path cell, the detection limit is about 6 µg/litre.[190] Arsine can also be passed into a heated graphite or quartz furnace mounted in an AAS instrument. The arsine can be continuously passed through the atomizer[191, 192] or collected in a cold trap and passed through rapidly when the cold trap in heated.[193, 194] This second technique provides the best detection limits which are in the fraction of a ng range.[195]

Neutron activation analysis is one of the more sensitive analytical methods. The arsenic-75 isotope is converted to arsenic-76 by thermal neutron absorption. Detection limits are near 1 ng, but the method is susceptible to interference. particularly from sodium. There have been many applications of this method in the analyses of biological samples,[196, 197, 198, 199] water[200] and particulate matter in air.[21] Activated sample solutions are frequently subjected to separation to eliminate 7m interfering radioisotopes.[201]

The determination of trace amounts of arsenic has also been performed using differential pulse polarography and anodic stripping voltametry.[202, 203, 204] The second of these methods was applied to biological samples that were wet ashed with nitric, sulfuric, and perchloric acids before distillation of arsenic as arsenic(III) chloride. The detection limit was in the ng range. Some of the organoarsenic compounds are also electroactive[205] but no practical methods for environmental analyses have appeared since mg/kg concentrations are required to observe responses.

A variety of other analytical methods have been successfully used for the determination of trace amounts of arsenic. Among these are: atomic emission spectroscopy,[206, 207, 208] x-ray fluorescence,[209] and isotope dilution mass spectrometry.[210]

An electron spectroscopic method (ESCA) has been reported in which arsine collected on filter surfaces was analysed.[211] Detection limits were in the ng range so that preconcentration resulted in further reduction of detection limits to sub µg/kg.

An enzyme method has been reported to give reasonable results in the 0.02–2.0 mg/kg range.[212]

II.2 Analyses for Specific Arsenic Compounds

Low concentrations of inorganic arsenic(III) and arsenic(V) in sea water can be determined using the molybdenum blue method.[186] Inorganic arsenic(III) and (V) can be separated by direct extraction with toluene of acidified aqueous solutions containing, for example, cysteine.[213] Differentiation between arsenic(III) and arsenic(V) is also possible using pH sensitive, selective reduction with sodium borohydride followed by atomic emission spectroscopy or AAS detection. Inorganic and methylarsenic compounds are reduced according to the reactions shown in Table II.1.

By buffering at pH 4, reduction of arsenic(V) is avoided. At pH 1.5, all compounds are reduced. The methylarsine compounds produced may be cold trapped, separated, and detected individually. Cold trapping and separation on heating, with detection by d.c. discharge in helium, has been used in the determination of arsenic in natural water, human urine[206, 214] and sea water[215, 31] at µg/kg and sub µg/kg concentrations. The detector cell has recently been studied and improved[216] as has the analysis train.[217]

Gas chromatographic detection of arsines trapped in cold toluene solvent using a microwave stimulated plasma detector has been developed by Talmi and Norvell.[218] The detection limits of this method are excellent (about 20 pg).

The electrochemical reactions of dimethylarsinic acid and trimethylarsine were studied by Eiton and Geiger.[205] Dimethylarsinic acid may be converted to its iodide and

Table II.1: Reduction Reactions of Inorganic and Methylarsenic Compounds

Compound	pka_1	pH	Product	B.P
Arsenous acid (meta) ($HAsO_2$)	9.23	< 7	AsH_3	−55°C
Arsenic acid (ortho) (H_3AsO_4)	2.20	> 4.0 1.5	No reaction AsH_3	−55°C
Methylarsonic acid [$CH_3AsO(OH)_2$]	4.1	> 5.0 1–5	Little reaction CH_3AsH_2	2°C
Dimethylarsenic acid [$(CH_3)_2AsO(OH)$]	6.2	1.5	$(CH_3)_2AsH$	36°C
Trimethylarsine oxid ($(CH_3)_3AsO$)	–	1.5	$(CH_3)_3As$	70°C
Phenylarsonic acid [$C_6H_5AsO(OH)_2$]	–	1.5	$C_6H_5AsH_2$	148°C
p-aminophenyl arsenic acid (arsanilic acid) $p-H_2N-C_6H_4AsO\,(OH)_2$	–	1.5	$H_3{}^+NC_6H_4\,AsH_2$	–

determined by gas chromatography[219] but the method is not applicable to the same wide range of arsenic compounds as the hydride-generating procedures.

Arsenic has been determined in marine organisms.[185] Substantial efforts have been made to identify the different organic arsenic compounds and, only recently, arsenobetaine was identified in rock lobsters[220] and arsenophospholipids in algae. Analytical methods for the determination of these compounds are not well developed. Thin layer chromatography was used in studies by Lunde,[222] the results of which indicated the possible presence of several as yet unidentified organic arsenic compounds.

Analytical methods for the determination of total arsenic and different forms of arsenic in human biological materials have been reviewed by Lauwerys *et al.*[213]

II.3 Some Interesting Studies on Arsenic Analysis

An acceptable analytical method for As (III) in groundwater must contend with other arsenic species as well as a number of other interferences. The arsenic species that are present in environmental samples are the inorganic species. As(III) and As (V), and the organic species, monomethylarsonic acid (MMA) and dimethylarsinic acid (DMA). The presence of other arsenic-containing species such as trimethylarsine oxide, monomethyl, dimethyl and trimethyl arsine, and arsenobetaine has not been reported in terrestrial or marine water.[223] Inorganic arsenic species are converted into the methylated forms of arsenic in the environment, and it has been reported that DMA is the predominant methylated species both in freshwater and seawater.[224]

$$O$$
$$\|$$
$$As$$
$$|$$
$$OH$$

As(III)
Arsenious acid

$$O$$
$$\|$$
$$HO - As - OH$$
$$|$$
$$OH$$

As(V)
Arsenic acid

$$O$$
$$\|$$
$$HO - As - OH$$
$$|$$
$$CH_3$$

Monomethylarsonic acid
(MMA)

$$O$$
$$\|$$
$$HO - As - CH_3$$
$$|$$
$$CH_3$$

Dimethylarsinic acid
(DMA)

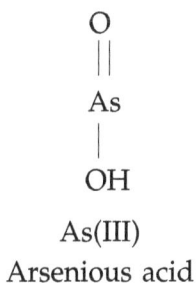

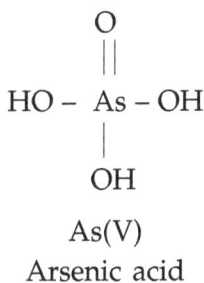

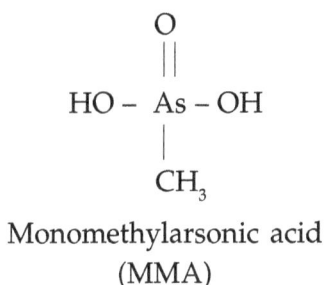

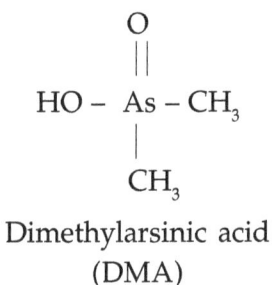

A knowledge of the concentration of these inorganic and organic arsenic species in aquatic systems may be important in understanding the transport of arsenic and the biochemical processes that involve arsenic species in these systems.

There is an abundant and often contradictory literature on the analysis of arsenic species in the environment. Of all the methods that have been proposed for the determination of the concentration of each of these organic and inorganic arsenic species at parts per billion levels, the most important and widely used methods are based on the conversion of each of these species into a volatile hydride followed by atomic absorption spectrophotometry (AAS). The absorbance of atomic arsenic is measured at 193.7 nm, or at the less sensitive arsenic resonance line at 197.2 nm. The separation methods that have been described for the four arsenic species include various chromatographic techniques such as electrophoresis, gas chromatography (GC), and high pressure liquid chromatography (HPLC). The most promising method of separation is based on an ion exchange technique. The following overview focuses the analytical methodology on arsenic determinations based on hydride generation and the separation of arsenic species based on ion exchange.

Yamamoto[225] described a method for the separation of arsenic (V), MMA, and DMA on a cation exchange column (Dowex 50 W–X8) into three fractions of eluted solution containing the three separated species. Each of the three fractions was digested with H_2SO_4 in a Kjeldahl flask. The arsenic species were reduced with Sn and HC1 to arsine. followed by the absorption of the arsine in a solution containing silver diethyldithiocarbamate and measurement of the absorbance of the resulting solution at 520 nm.[226] It should be noted that only the three arsenic species, As(V), MMA, and DMA, can be separated by use of cation exchange resin.

The sensitivity of the method described by Yamamoto is limited by the sensitivity of the spectrophotometric method employed for the determination of the arsine that is volatilized from solution. This spectrophotometric method has been, for many years, the recommended method for the determination of total inorganic arsenic. As(III), and As(V), in water and waste water.[227] The method has been modified for the determination of As (III) by the addition of dimethylformamide to prevent the reduction of As(V) to AsH_3.[228] This recommended method can also be used for the determination of one of the organic arsenic species, MMA, because MMA can be reduced to methylarsine which, like arsine, forms a colored reaction product with silver diethyldithiocarbamate. The absorption bands of the two reaction products are well separated (by about 40 nm) in the visible region and therefore MMA can also be determined by the recommended spectrophotometric method. The presence of DMA, however, interferes with this determination.[229]

Zinc-HCl is a stronger reducing agent that Sn-HCl and, therefore, both reducing agents are able to readily reduce As(V) as well as As(III) to AsH_3. A mixture of sodium borohydride ($NaBH_4$) and HC1 was also found to be an effective reducing agent for the generation of AsH_3 from As(V) or As(III).[230, 231] The implication was that none of the three reducing agents could differentiate between As(III) and As(V) in solution. It is known, however, that the reduction potential of the As(V) → As (III) couple decreases with increasing pH and, because multi-electron transfer reactions are often slow, the two electron reduction, As(V) → As(III), is expected to be slower at high pH than at low pH. Based on this phenomena, it is possible to determine As (III) and As(V) in a mixture by controlling the pH at which $NaBH_4$ converts the arsenic species to AsH_3. If the pH of the solution is maintained between 4 and 5 in a mixture containing As(III) and As(V), only As(III) is converted to AsH_3 by $NaBH_4$. The total arsenic in solution can be determined because As(III) is converted to AsH_3, by $NaBH_4$. The total arsenic in solution can be determined because As(III) and As(V) are both converted into AsH_3 in 5 M HCl.[232, 233, 234] The measurement technique used by all these workers was AAS.

The volatilized hydrides can be determined quantitatively by (1) the recommended spectrophotometric method, (2) a gas chromatography-mass spectrometry method (GC-MS), or (3) an atomic absorption method. The spectrophotometric method lacks the sensitivity required for the determination of parts per billion levels of arsenic often required for groundwater. The GC-MS method has the necessary selectivity, but requires the use of an internal standard for the quantitative determination of a single species,[235] and a preliminary separation for the determination of parts per billion levels of As(III), As(V). MMA, and DMA in a large number of environmental or toxicological samples, the GC-MS method is, therefore, too elaborate and time consuming. It has been implied that a mixture of all four arsenic species can be determined quantitatively by kinetic control of the $NaBH_4$ reduction.[236] For routine analytical determinations, however, a preliminary separation must be performed. The four-component mixture must be separated into the individual constituents. either before or after the reduction process,[237] by condensation of the volatile hydrides in a cold trap followed by the selective volatilization of the solid hydrides.[233]

The analysis of mixtures containing the inorganic arsenic species As(III) and As(V) as well as the organic arsenic species, MMA and DMA, by the hydride generation technique is subject to errors caused by the presence of the methylated arsenic species. In a well-buffered solution at a pH in the vicinity of 5, As(III) can be determined with minimal interference by the presence of As(V); the presence of MMA and DMA, however, can give erroneous results because a small amount of hydride is generated from the MMA and a considerable amount is generated from the DMA. It has been suggested that the MMA is partially converted into species such as $CH_3As(OH)_2$, and that the DMA is present primarily as the undissociated form, $(CH_3)_2AsO(OH)$ ($pK_a = 6.2$), in the well-buffered solution at pH 5. These species of MMA and DMA are reactive and readily form volatile hydrides.[238] Similar interferences can be encountered when the hydride generation is carried out in 5 M HCl for the determination of As(V) in the presence of MMA and DMA. The MMA present is almost completely converted to the hydride and a small amount of the DMA is also volatilized as the hydride.[238] In the analysis of environmental samples containing the methylated species of arsenic, the hydride generation technique is best employed after carrying out a preliminary separation of the four-component mixture.

The ideal method for the quantitative determination of arsenic is the atomic absorption method; it is simple, rapid and convenient, and has the necessary sensitivity for the determination of parts per billion levels of arsenic. The conversion of the hydride to atomic arsenic has been accomplished in an air-entrained hydrogen-argon flame,[232] in a quartz tube heated with an air-acetylene flame,[239] or in a graphite tube.[223] It has been claimed that the use of an atomic emission technique, instead of the atomic absorption method, gives an increased sensitivity for the determination of arsenic. Indeed, both direct current plasmas[240, 241] and inductively coupled plasmas[242, 243] have been used for the measurement of atomic arsenic emission.

II.3.1 Determination of Arsenic by Hydride Generation and Atomic Absorption Spectrophotometry

Most of the conflicting results reported on the determination of arsenic by the hydride generation method with $NaBH_4$ can be attributed to variations in the production of the hydride and its transport into the atomizer, which is a flame, plasma, graphite furnace, or heated quartz tube. Several investigations of the factors that control hydride production have shown that it is important to optimize a number of variables for each configuration of the hydride generation equipment. A simple hydride generator can be assembled, as shown in Figure II.1. A 100 ml three-neck round bottom flask is fitted with a drain tube and a stopcock, and one neck of the flask is fitted with a stopper into which a glass plunger is inserted. The plunger is a convenient means for the introduction of a pellet of $NaBH_4$ into the solution in the hydride generator. Alternatively, a rubber septum can be fitted over one neck of the flask and a syringe containing a solution of $NaBH_4$ in NaOH can be injected. Nitrogen gas is bubbled through a sintered glass frit at the end of a tube that is inserted through the top neck of the hydride generator. The third neck of the hydride generator, fitted with a rubber septum, is used to introduce the sample solution into the generator. The generated arsine gas is swept out through the exit tube in the top neck of the generator and collected in a cold trap with liquid nitrogen. The use of a nitrogen- or argon-entrained air-hydrogen flame gives excellent sensitivity for routine arsenic determination. The absorbance vs. time profiles or peak shapes are dependent on a number of factors that include the stability of the gaseous hydride, the solubility of the hydride in the solution in the generator,

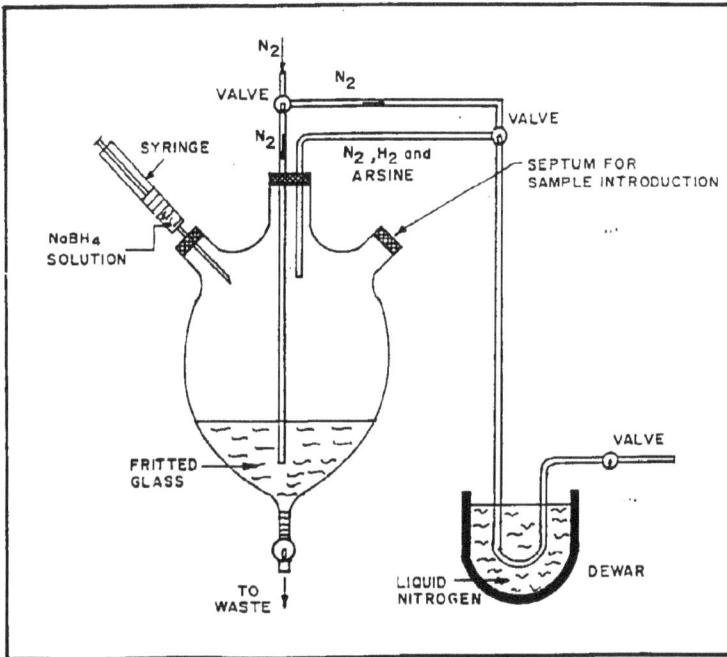

Figure II.1: Hydride Generator Assembly

the acidity and the temperature of this solution, the carrier gas flow rate, the rate of hydrogen gas evolution in the hydride generator, the amount of $NaBH_4$ added, and the temperature of the flame (or atomizer). The peak heights of these absorbance vs. time profiles can be used to determine arsenic concentrations in the range 1.7 to 100 ppb. An increase in sensitivity and a significant improvement in the reproducibility are obtained if the evolved arsine is condensed in a cold trap and released instantaneously into the atomizer. If this cold trap procedure is employed, the $NaBH_4$ reduction can be performed over a longer time to ensure complete reduction by the addition of several aliquots of the $NaBH_4$ solution to the reaction mixture.[234, 244]

The efficiency of the hydride generation reaction is reduced in the presence of ions that consume the reductant, *e.g.*, cations such as Ag(I), Fe(III), Au(III), Pt(IV), Sb(III). and Sn(II) and anions such as F⁻ and S^{-2} interfere with the hydride generation reaction. The effect of these interferences may be minimized by the addition of appropriate masking agents.[245] Investigators have also reported that transition metal ions such as Co (II) and Ni(II) severely interfere with the determination of arsenic by the hydride generation technique.[246] The mechanism of these interfering cations and anions has been discussed extensively. It has been suggested that the interference is caused by the precipitation of the interfering element in a finely divided form which adsorbs the evolved arsine gas and subsequently decomposes it.[247, 249] An alternative explanation is that a soluble species is formed between the interfering species and the AsH_3. The arsine that is combined in this manner can be regenerated from the same solution by the addition of a masking agent and $NaBH_4$ solution.[250]

Various chelating agents mask the interferences caused by the presence of transition metal ions. The chelating agents or masking agents that have been recommended are EDTA. pyridine-2-aldoxine, and 2,2'-dipyridyl.[251] One of the more effective reagents that has been used to minimize the interference from transition metals is L-cystine, in which the disulfide group is easily reduced and kinetically favoured over the reduction of a transition metal ion to its elemental state. The use of a 3 per cent solution of L-cystine in 5 M HC1 eliminated the interference by a number of transition metals in the generation of AsH_3, from As(III) and As(V).[252]

In situations where the hydride generation technique gives non-reproducible results for one or more reasons described above, a flameless atomic absorption method can be employed by using a graphite furnace. A matrix modifier, such as a solution of nickel nitrate or a mixture of nickel nitrate and nitric acid, is added to the sample solution containing one of the four arsenic species. The solution is introduced into the graphite furnace in which As(V), As(III), MMA, or DMA is converted into arsenic atoms and the atomic absorption is measured at an arsenic resonance line.[253] The addition of nickel nitrate as a matrix modifier probably forms nonvolatile nickel arsenides in the graphite furnace thereby stabilizing the As in the graphite tube, allowing higher temperatures to be used for drying and charring which leads to cleaner and more reproducible atomization.[254]

II.3.2 Ion Exchange Chromatography

It has become evident from the conflicting results reported in the literature that the determination of trace levels of As (III), As(V), MMA, and DMA in environmental samples is difficult and subject to a number of interferences. A method that has given consistently reliable results is based on a preliminary separation of the four components followed by the conversion of each of the components into a volatile hydride and subsequently into arsenic atoms which are determined by atomic absorption (or emission) spectrophotometry. The preliminary separation is accomplished by ion exchange chromatography. Three of the arsenic species. As(V), MMA, and DMA, can be conveniently separated on a cation exchange column (Dowex 50 W–X8).[225] A 10 ml solution (pH $\leq$ 2) containing

10 µg As/ml was added to the cation exchange column (32 cm long and 1 cm diameter), and the column was eluted successively with 40 ml of 0.2 M trichloroacetic acid (pH ≤ 1), 30 ml of 1.8 M sodium acetate, and 50 ml of 1.0 M sodium hydroxide (pH > 12) at an elution rate of about 1 ml/min. Three fractions were collected; the first 25 ml fraction contained the As(V), the next 45 ml fraction contained the MMA and the DMA was eluted in the final 50 ml fraction. A modification of this separation technique gave more reproducible results. The cation exchange column (30 cm × 1 cm I.D.) was packed with the cation exchange resin (AG 50 W–X8) and conditioned with 50 ml of 1 M NH_3, 70 ml of 1 M HCl, and 30 ml of 0.5 M HCl before use, so that the pH in the column was < 1.5. The sample solution (2 ml containing 1 to 5 µg As) at pH < 2 was added to the top of the column and eluted with 30 ml of 0.2 M trichloroacetic acid followed by 70 ml of 1 M ammonium acetate, and 5 ml fractions of the effluent were collected and analyzed in a graphite atomizer by flameless AAS. A matrix modification method was employed because the atomic absorption signal obtained with As(V), MMA, and DMA differed significantly in standards containing the same amount of As. The addition of nickel nitrate to the sample solution as a matrix modifier, before it was introduced into the graphite furnace, stabilized the signal from the three arsenic species. It was found that the first 20 ml of the effluent from the cation exchange column contained the As(V), the next 40 ml contained the MMA, and the DMA was eluted in the final 40 ml. The use of the cation exchange resin as described above, by Yamamoto[225] and modified by Iverson *et al.*[225] resulted in the separation of the three arsenic

species. As (V), MMA, and DMA. All four arsenic-containing species were determined by combining a digestion and reduction scheme with ion-exchange chromatography,[256] and the concentration of As (V) was determined by difference; the method, however, is much too laborious and time consuming for routine use.

Another approach resulted in the separation of all four arsenic species on a single column containing both cation and anion-exchange resins. The concentration of arsenic in each eluted fraction was determined by flameless AAS. A solution of nitric acid and nickel nitrate was added as a matrix modifier to each sample solution.[237] The chromatographic column (35 cm × 1 cm I.D.) was packed with 9 cm of an anion exchange resin (AG1–X8), followed by 26 cm of a cation exchange resin (AG 50 W–X8), and washed several times, successively, with 70 ml of each of the following solutions: 1.5 M NH_3, 1 M HCl, and 0.48 M HCl at a flow rate of 5 to 10 ml/min. The sample (2 ml containing 0.08 to 4 µg total As), was added to the top of the column and eluted with 55 ml of 0.006 M trichloroacetic acid (at 2 ml/min), followed by 8 ml of 0.2 M trichloroacetic acid (at 2ml/min), 55 ml of 1.5 M NH_3 (at 6 ml/min) and finally, 50 ml of 0.2 M trichloroacetic acid (at 6 ml/min). The eluted fractions (3 to 20 ml) were collected, treated with the nickel matrix modification solution, and analyzed by the flameless atomic absorption method.

The acid dissociation constants of the four arsenic species demonstrate why ion exchange chromatography is an effective separation method. Approximate values for the pKa's of the four arsenic species are

	pK_1	pK_2	pK_3
As(III) : Arsenious acid	9.2	–	–
As(V) : Arsenic acid	2.2	6.9	11.5
(MMA) : Monomethylarsonic acid	4.1	8.7	–
(DMA) : Dimethylarsinic acid	1.6	6.3	–

At pH $\approx$ 2.5 (in 0.006 M trichloroacetic acid), the As(III) exists in solution as a neutral species, and the As(V) exists primarily as an anionic species; at this pH, the MMA and DMA are also mostly in their neutral forms. The As (V), therefore, has a high affinity for an anion exchange resin, whereas the As(III), MMA, and DMA are not retained, at this pH, on the anion exchange column. The 55 ml of the 0.0006 M trichloroacetic acid therefore strips the neutral As(III) species from both the cation and the anion exchange resins and elutes it in the first 23 ml of the eluted solution, while the negatively charged As(V) species is strongly retained on the anion exchange resin. The addition of 8 ml of 0.2 M trichloroacetic acid lowers the pH to less than 1.0. This converts all the MMA in solution to its neutral form and the DMA is protonated and retained strongly on the cation exchange resin. The second fraction of the eluted solution (23 to 55 ml). therefore, contains the MMA. The resin column now contains the As(V) species strongly bound on the anion exchange resin and the DMA species strongly bound on the cation exchange resin. As the more concentrated trichloroacetic acid solution (pH < 1.0) enters the anion exchange resin bed (at the bottom of the resin column), and As (V) is converted into its neutral form and is collected in the third fraction of the eluted solution (55 to 85 ml). The only arsenic species left in the chromatographic column is the cationic form of DMA, which is strongly bound to the cation exchange resin. Addition of the solution of 1.5 M NH_3 (pH $\approx$ 12) converts the DMA into its anionic form, strips it from the cation exchange resin at the top of the chromatographic column, carries it into the anion exchange resin at the top of the chromatographic column, and then carries it into the anion exchange resin at the bottom of the column where it is strongly retained. Finally, the addition of 0.2 M trichloroacetic acid protonates the anionic DMA species and elutes it from the bottom of the chromatographic column in the final fraction of the eluted solution (135 to 175 ml). This elution order may be followed by reference to Figure II.2 in which the fractional concentrations of the arsenic species present in solutions of the As(III), As(V), MMA, and DMA are plotted as a function of pH. The separation of the four arsenic species is rationalized on the basis of their acid dissociation constants, but it must be recognized that non-polar interactions occur between the solute species and the resins, and in this instance these interactions are assumed to be weak.[257].

II.3.3 Recommended Method for the Determination of Arsenic Species in Groundwater

Before embarking on an analysis of the arsenic species, it is essential to determine whether the groundwater is heavily contaminated, especially with metal ions or organic matter. In such instances, a preliminary wet digestion procedure should be used before separation of the arsenic species, but care must be taken to avoid losses caused by volatilization and the oxidation of As (III) to As(V). The concentrations of the four arsenic species that are found in most groundwater supplies can be determined by performing a preliminary ion chromatographic separation,

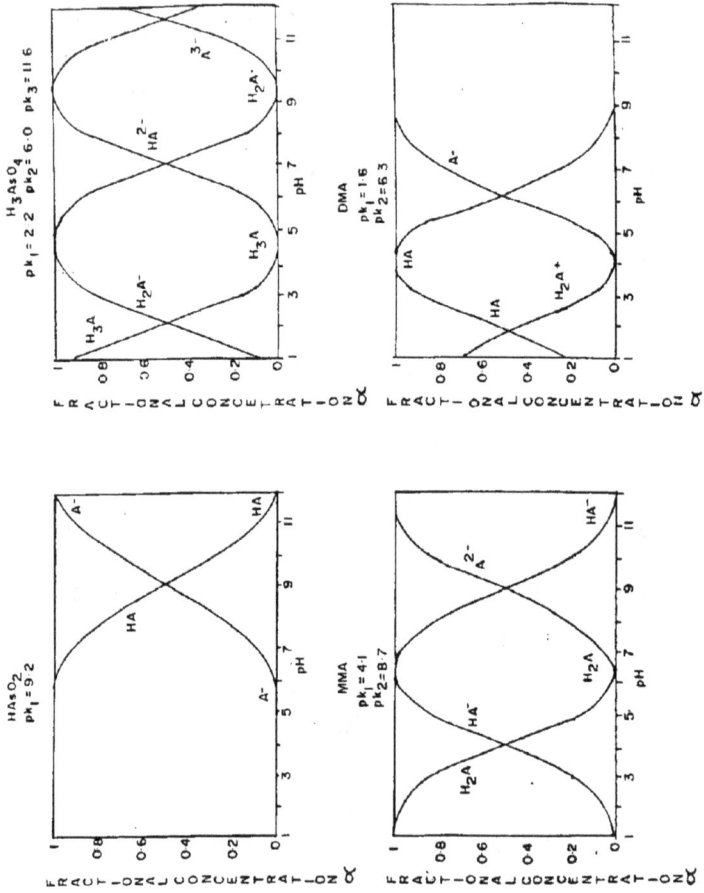

Figure II.2: Fractional Concentration of Arsenic Species Plotted as a Function of pH

as described above, on a column packed with an anion exchange resin and a cation exchange resin. The arsenic content in the four fractions that are collected can be determined by flameless AAS after addition of the nickel matrix modifier to each fraction. Alternatively, in the absence of interfering ions in solution, the hydride flame atomic absorption method can be employed. The fractions containing the As(III) and the As(V) are analyzed by the hydride generation technique by the addition of $NaBH_4$ in 5 M HCl. The fractions containing the MMA and DMA are wet digested with H_2SO_4 and then converted into the volatile hydride by the addition of $NaBH_4$.

Need for Development of Arsenic Testing Field Kit

A major problem related to the availability of potable water for millions of people in rural regions of West Bengal and Bangladesh concerns the lack of civil infrastructure for selection, screening, testing and monitoring ground water samples for arsenic concentration levels. Such testing and monitoring will contribute significantly to the public health and safety of people who inhabit regions where aquifers are contaminated by arsenic.

Recognizing the enormity and severity of the problem of arsenic poisoning, the capabilities of commercially available arsenic detection filed kits were critically evaluated both in the laboratory and in the arsenic affected areas in West Bengal, India and Bangladesh for their accuracy.[271] The detection limits of these kits are different and accordingly their utility will depend on the specific purpose, which they are intended to serve. Some of the kits have no provision for elimination of sulphide interference in the estimation of arsenic. When these studies were carried out, none of the kits available in India and Bangladesh in its present form, was capable of detecting arsenic concentration as low as 0.01 mg/L or 10 μg/L, the recommended WHO guideline value for arsenic in drinking water.

In the backdrop of the evaluation of the arsenic detection field kits their merits and limitations, an urgent need was felt to develop a simple, accurate, prudent, user friendly, indigenous field kit which can be used for rapid on-site screening of arsenic contaminated water sources; free from most of the limitations experienced in commercially available arsenic detection field kits and capable of detecting arsenic concentration as low as 0.01 mg/L, the guideline value set by WHO for arsenic. A prototype unit has been developed by NEERI which meets most of the requirements of an ideal field kit for arsenic[272] (Plates 3–6).

Annexure III
R&D Projects on Arsenic in India (Year 1997)

III.0.1. Organisation

University of Kalyani, Faculty of Science, Department of Chemistry, Kalyani – 741 235 (W.B.)

Project Title

Mechanism of mobilisation of arsenic in sedimentary aquifers in West Bengal and realistic approaches for *in situ* remediation methods.

Objectives

The proposed objectives have been divided under two parts such as short-term and long-term goals.

Short-term Goals

1. Systematic sedimentary petrological investigations for provance determination.

2. To investigate the level of pH, E_h, DO in selective wells to understand the redox condition.

3. To investigate the impacts of anthropogenic inputs responsible for arsenic mobilisation–laboratory, designed stimulated experiments with varying influencing factors.

4. To investigate the effects of artificial recharging test (pond as well as tank system pilot scale experiments) to restrict the mobilisation of arsenic from sediment to groundwater.

5. Design of low-cost filter unit(s)/field model(s) for removal of arsenic both on-site/off-site. The performances of the unit/model would be evaluated in the light of technical and economic feasibility.

6. To study the safe disposal of sludge containing high arsenic.

Long-term Goals

1. To carry out hydrogeological study to explore the causative factors of spreading of arsenic vertically as well as laterally and prediction of safer zone for trapping arsenic free groundwater.

2. To investigate the sealing mechanism and development of low-cost technique to prevent downward movement of arsenic rich water.

3. To understand the impact of land use pattern for arsenic mobilisation and possible mitigation options.

Scope of Work

Sedimentological Investigation

The major task that would be carried out:

(a) Identification of source terrain for individual sedimentary packages;

(b) Clay mineralogy of the argillic sediments;

(c) Diagenetic approach for the process responsible for the formation of sulphide (S^{--}) phases, mainly Fe/As–sulphides under reducing conditions;

(d) S-isotopic studies in order to characterise the genetic source of sulphur in sediments.

Redox Measurement

In-situ measurement of pH, E_h and DO to understand the arsenic speciation as well as transformation for the mobilisation of arsenic from sediment to groundwater. Selective extraction using oxalate and pyrophosphate media to understand the role of As with the secondary Fe, Al and Mn phases as well as the organic carbon.

Arsenic Mobilisation Laboratory Tests

Laboratory based E_h–pH measurement in fresh sediments under the variable NO_3, PO_4 and free carbon loading rate to understand the mobilisation of arsenic from sediment to groundwater.

Artificial Recharging Test

Pilot scale artificial recharging test in Chakdaha block of Nadia District based on data/information of the local geohydrological conditions. Lysimeter studies would be conducted to monitor the chemistry of the infiltrating water.

Design of Filter Unit/Model

Laboratory experiments for the selection of suitable low-cost geochemical material for the removal technique. Bench scale study for the selection of design parameters. On site testing of the field model/field test of the filter unit based on optimised design parameters developed in the bench scale study. Full scale field tests of the model/filter unit. Construction as well as fabrication of cost effective commercial filter units for the users with the help of PHED, Govt. of West Bengal.

Safe disposal of sludge *i.e.* bio-degradability study to convert harmless form of arsenical compounds.

Time Frame and Budgetary Estimate

The project will be phased over a period of three years (1st year–Phase-I, 2nd year–Phase-II, 3rd year–Phase III).

Budget (Year 1997)   **in Rs.'000**

	1st Year	2nd Year	3rd Year
A. Recurring grant	932	715	359
B. Non-recurring grant (Equipment)	554	54	
Total (A+B) Rs. 26.14 lakhs			

Progress/Achievement

The arsenic containing groundwater in West Bengal occurs in sediments formed by meandering rivers. From place to place the sediments differ, hydrochemistry varies and with that the concentration of arsenic. Arsenic containing pyrite and arsenopyrites in association with ferric hydroxides is found in the more clayey sediments.

Two possible mechanisms for the release of arsenic to ground.water have been visualised:

Mechanism-1

An anaerobic environment is exposed to oxygen rich groundwater which leads to dissolve arsenic and ferrous ions in the water due to weathering

Mechanism-2

In an aerobic environment iron can be oxidised and precipitated as ferric hydroxide. On the surface of ferric hydroxide arsenic is adsorbed. During an aerobic condition the iron is reduced to Fe^{2+} and arsenic is released. Phosphorous is also released by the same mechanism.

Arsenic chemistry of groundwater extracted from several wells indicate the varying ratio of As(V)/As(III) species. Scrutiny of the preliminary data reveals that As-mobilisation in the groundwater is related to reduction of As-species commonly absorbed on the secondary Fe and Al-phases. The high As-concentration is generally associated with high Fe-concentration and the nature of groundwater is normally alkaline to acidic. The water quality monitoring shows low chloride and sulphate but high phosphate and nitrate. Thus, the groundwater in West Bengal are low in sulphate *i.e.* not oxygen rich, which makes the Mechanism-1 less likely. Elevated phosphate contents support the Mechanism-2 inferring that Ferric Oxide/ Hydroxide are reduced to soluble ferrous iron. E_h-pH field and laboratory data also established the reduction of Fe^{3+} to Fe^{2+} with positive co-relation with free carbon and p-block element.

III.0.2 Organisation

National Metallurgical Laboratory, Jamshedpur–831 007.

Project Title

Development of a low cost filtering medium for the removal of arsenic from ground water.

Objectives of the Study

(a) *Primary objective*

The primary objective is to develop a filtering medium which will be able to remove arsenic from groundwater by a single filter operation. The operation will involve no pre-filter or post-filter treatment of the groundwater. The filtering medium will be made available in the form of candles/pellets/powder. The filter will be low cost and well within the means of the low income rural population.

(b) *Secondary objective*

As a prerequisite for obtaining the primary objective, following secondary objectives have been identified.

- ✮ Identification of the right raw material
- ✮ Treatment of the raw material to get the desired property.
- ✮ A thorough appraisal of the arsenic and allied elemental concentrations in the water, soil and plant samples of the places under study.
- ✮ Development of an analytical technique for quick and accurate analysis of arsenic samples.
- ✮ Development of a spot analytical technique for the screening of arsenic samples at the site.

Scope and Coverage

Arsenic catastrophe in West Bengal is biggest of its own kind in the world. About 30 million people spread over an area of 3000 sq.km. covering six districts are struggling to cope up with the arsenic menace. As of now about a million people are regularly consuming arsenic contaminated water and about 2 million people are showing arsenic related skin problems in addition to other ailments. The vegetation and the domestic animals are also being affected as their water need is primarily supported by the groundwater. For example, cow milk in the affected areas is showing higher levels of arsenic than it actually consumes through water. It is imperative that unless immediate remedial steps are taken, the tragedy is going to strike in an unprecedented manner.

Majority of the people suffering from arsenic contamination hail from rural Bengal. They depend mostly on agriculture for their livelihood. It is beyond their means to adopt any expensive measure for water purification. Provision of a public water distribution network at the government level also seems to be a remote possibility.

It is with this perspective that the present work is most pertinent. People should be provided with some method to purify water at domestic level well within their means. Present work aims at developing a filtering medium in the form of powder/pellet/candle for removing arsenic from groundwater. The material will be essentially a treated clay and the production cost will be essentially[1] a treated clay and the production cost will also be low. The product will be ideally suitable for the lower income group. Further, the proposed filtering operation will be one stage, will not involve any sophisticated arrangement and may be accomplished with household utensils or earthen pots. There will not be any need for a pre-filter and post-filter treatment of the water.

This work has been conceived and planned with reference to the arsenic problem in West Bengal. However, the study is general in nature and the filtering material may be used anywhere and for any water sample containing arsenic.

The primarily monitorable output in the present work is the arsenic concentration before and after the filtration. However, other parameters like, pH, other metal concentrations hardness, anion concentrations and other allied parameters which make the water potable will also be monitored.

Time Frame

One year.

Budgetary Estimate (Year 1997)

Rs. 3.304 lakhs (Rupees three lakhs thirty thousand and four hundred only)

Progress Achieved

☆ The project has been completed on schedule

☆ Two low cost materials have been developed which are good adsorbents for both As(III) and As (V)

☆ Blending studies have been performed to make these materials suitable for making water filter candles

☆ Application is being prepared to patent one of these materials

☆ Completion report has been written and will be forwarded to RGNDWM shortly.

III.0.3 Organisation

Centre for Study of Man and Environment, Kolkata – 700 091

Project Title

Geology and geochemistry of arsenic occurrences in groundwater of six districts of West Bengal.

Progress Report

Arsenic occurs in ground water of 6 districts of West Bengal at above permissible limit (0.05 mg/l) putting 1 million people under risk affecting few of them dermatologically. Important findings regarding arsenic occurrences in West Bengal are as follows:

1. It occurs in places in the groundwater of rural sectors of the affected districts. Intensive agriculture is common land use practice of the area with ground water as the major source of irrigation.

2. The lithologic succession of the area is mainly loose alluvial sands of late Quaternary age with intercalations of clay. Arsenic occurs mainly in the waters tapping from shallower aquifers (<100 m depth). At present the occurrence of arsenic in waters tapping from deeper aquifers (>100 m depth) is rare.

3. All waters tapping from similar depths of same aquifer are not arsenious. Even within tens of metre, one tube well yields arsenious water with concentration as high as 0.4 mg/l while the other yields arsenic free water.

4. There exist strong positive correlations between arsenic (alkali digested) and extractable Cu, Pb, Fe, Mn of the sediments.

5. Concentration of As in the argillaceous sediments are higher than that of arsenaceous sediments. It ranges between 2 and 8 ppm in the former while bdl and 3 ppm in the later.

6. Heavy minerals assemblage of these sediments in order of abundance are garnet–kyanite–hornblende–staurolite–sillimanite–opaques–biotite–chlorite–tourmaline–epidote.

7. XRD analysis reveals that the clays are dominantly of illitic type.

8. Arsenic occurs in ground water mostly in trivalent state.

III.0.4 Organisation

School of Environmental Studies (SOES), Jadavpur University, Kolkata.

Project Title

Biotransformation and sink of arsenic from groundwater by microalgal based biotreatment system.

Progress Report

The present study was undertaken in 1996 to develop a cost-effective safe microalgal based arsenic removal system. So far six freshwater microalgal system have been tested in-vivo at different levels of arsenic concentrations (*i.e.* 0.25 mg/l, 0.1 to 1 mg/l and 1 to 20 mg/l). The optimum cultural conditions, growth rate of the organisms, metal removal efficiency, determination of cellular bound arsenic contents etc. were measured in each test systems.

Microalgal biotreatment system for removal of arsenic from contaminated water was attempted over past one year. Several microalgal test organisms were tested so far at both lower (0.1 to 1 mg/l) and higher (1 to 20 mg/l) concentration of arsenic contaminated systems separately. The details of the observation of the present study is given in Table III.1. From the present study it appears that the most efficient system was the mixed algal culture of *Oscillatoria* and *Lyngbia* and this is followed by *Euglena gracilis* and *Scenedesmus bijuga* system separately. The efficiency of the removal was measured at an interval of 7 days upto 21st days of treatment. However, the days of treatment can be reduced with increasing the treatment innoculum load of each test algae. These conditions have to be standardised in open *in vivo* system.

It is further interesting to note the fact that the more than 95 per cent of the metal was accumulated in the cytoplasm rather than bound to cell wall (Table III.2). From the cytoplasm, the cell may biotransform the same into organic form like MMA and DMA as reported earlier by Maeda *et al.*

Thus the microbial removal of arsenic contamination particularly by photo-autotrophic organisms like algae may have some limitation in field application as the process appears to be bit slower than any chemical treatment

Table III.1: Arsenic Removal Efficiency by Various Microalgae

Sl.No.	Test Algae	Arsenic No. Concentration Range (mg/L)	Maximum Arsenic Removal (Per cent) Under Different Period of Incubation		
			7 Days	14 Days	21 Days
1.	Scenedesmus bijuga	Lower	30	37	38
		Higher	14	48	51
2.	Ankistrodesmus convolutua	Lower	20	30	35
		Higher	18	32	45
3.	Euglena gracilis	Lower	15	28	50
		Higher	24	30	60
4.	Spirulina platensis	Lower	10	20	40
		Higher	18	32	45
5.	Mixed culture of Oscillatoria sp. and Lyngbia sp.	Lower	42	48	60
		Higher	31	47	53

Lower: 0.1 to 1 mg/l; Higher: 1 to 20 mg/l.

system. However, it will be an addition support in safe transformed forms (*i.e.* methylation of inorganic arsenic forms). Thus combined treatment facilities may be an ideal choice for tackling the problem for supplying arsenic free drinking water.

Table III.2: Localisation of Arsenic (Per cent) in Cellular Components of Test Organisms

Sl.No.	Test Organism	Per cent Localised in Cellular Component	
		Cytoplasm	Cellwall
1.	Scenedesmus bijuga	96.5	3.5
2.	Ankistrodesmus convolutes	93.5	6.5
3.	Euglena gracilis	85.0	15.0
4.	Spirulina platensis	95.5	4.5
5.	Mixed algae of Oscillatoria and Lyngbia	91.5	9.5

III.0.5 Organisation

School of Environmental Studies (SOES), Jadavpur University, Kolkata

Project Title

Arsenic species along with other metal/metalloid present and responsible for the Arsenic Episode in groundwater of West Bengal and a cheap technique to remove arsenic, thus making the ground water suitable for drinking and cooking.

Progress Report

Since 1978, time to time reports of arsenic contamination in ground water and suffering of people in some districts of the state of West Bengal, India, due to drinking arsenic contaminated water were reported. Till 1988, practically no attention was given on this problem about the source of arsenic and the population affected drinking the contaminated water. A number of hypotheses have been put forward as regards to the probable source of arsenic that contaminating the ground water. These are (*i*) tube-well filters, (*ii*) pesticides and insecticides, (*iii*) fertilisers (*iv*) arsenic containing materials dumped underground during last world war. However none of the above hypotheses would be consistent with physical evidence. A systematic study by Jadavpur University team for the first time reveals that the amount of arsenic withdrawn from underground by a single Municipal Water Supply Scheme supplying water in a few villages alone comes to about 150 kg. of arsenic per year and out of that about 50 per cent is As(III) and 50 per cent As(V). Again no methyl or dimethyl arsenic acid could be found in ground water. Thus the source of arsenic is expected to be geological.

The six districts of West Bengal affected are Nadia, Murshidabad, Malda, Bardhaman, 24 Parganas (North), 24 Parganas (South). The total geographical area and population of West Bengal are 88,752 sq.km. and 67 millions respectively. Total area and population of these affected six districts are respectively 34,000 sq.km. and 30 millions. Total population and area where we surveyed till August, 1992, and could find arsenic are 2.8 millions and 4,000 sq.km. respectively. It may be mentioned that all the people of the area where we found arsenic are not arsenic affected and drinking arsenic contaminated water. Arsenic is not found in all tube-wells and all depths. Around 500,000 (five hundred thousand) people within the area we have sampled are showing the manifestation related to arsenic toxicity (pigementary changes, arsenical keratoses etc.) and arsenic concentration in hair, nail, urine, scales to the affected people are very high. We believe more we will survey in these districts more areas and arsenic affected people will be found. So far we have analysed water samples at about 900 different locations in these six districts and out of that in about 650 samples we have found arsenic. The range of arsenic in these tube-wells are from above maximum permissible limit (0.05 mg/l) to 3.5 mg/l. The average value is 0.25 mg/l. The recommended value in drinking water is 0.01 mg/l. From the results of our study for last 3 years more than 20,000 school children in these six districts are drinking arsenic contaminated water and eight Municipal Water Supply Schemes in these six districts distributing more than 1.0 million gallon of water/day to the villages and water contain arsenic in the range 0.1– 0.54 ppm.

We could not find arsenic above the maximum permissible value in surface water and surface well around 30–40 ft. deep. So the possibility of geological source is expected. To establish this fact we analysed arsenic at different depths bore–hole soil samples in these six districts. In one set of soil samples out of the five different bore–hole soils in these districts we could hit a layer at 260–290 ft. which contains elevated amount of arsenic. We analysed bore–hole soil samples at each 10 ft. depth. From surface layer till 260 ft. we found arsenic in the range 0.1–3.0 ppm. At 260–270, 270–280, 280–290 ft. the arsenic content in the soil/rock suddenly increased to 18 ppm, 42 ppm and 22 ppm respectively. After 290 ft. till 330 ft. the arsenic content is less than 1.0 ppm. These three layers 260– 290 ft. are different in nature from rest of the soil samples. The reason why arsenic is leaching out from underground soil/ rock is not clear, however, it may be due to some geo–chemical reactions inside what may be the result of heavy water withdrawal from under ground for irrigation. In all these six districts water demands of almost 100 per cent are met from underground sources (irrigation, water supply, schemes and domestic use).

Since these villagers are not using any alternative water source other than ground water, they are drinking arsenic contaminated water. To supply the villagers arsenic free water for drinking and cooking the Jadavpur University research team has developed a filter which along with one tablet (chemical compound) and two locally made earthen-jars could remove almost 100 per cent of the arsenic from the contaminated water. The system is suitable for supplying, 10–20 liters good quality arsenic-free drinking water daily. The cost of the whole system for one year use will be rupees one hundred twenty (four US $ approx) only.

From our studies made during the last 3 years in these six districts, it has become clear that if no alternative water is made available to the people and no control measures taken to provide arsenic free drinking water these regions may turn into graveyard in not so distant future. We also feel, the elevated arsenic in ground water may not be restricted only in these six districts and also in state West Bengal alone.

The map of the affected blocks of the six districts is given in Figure III.1. Table III.3 shows some data on affected districts. Figure III.2 shows the filtering apparatus. Table

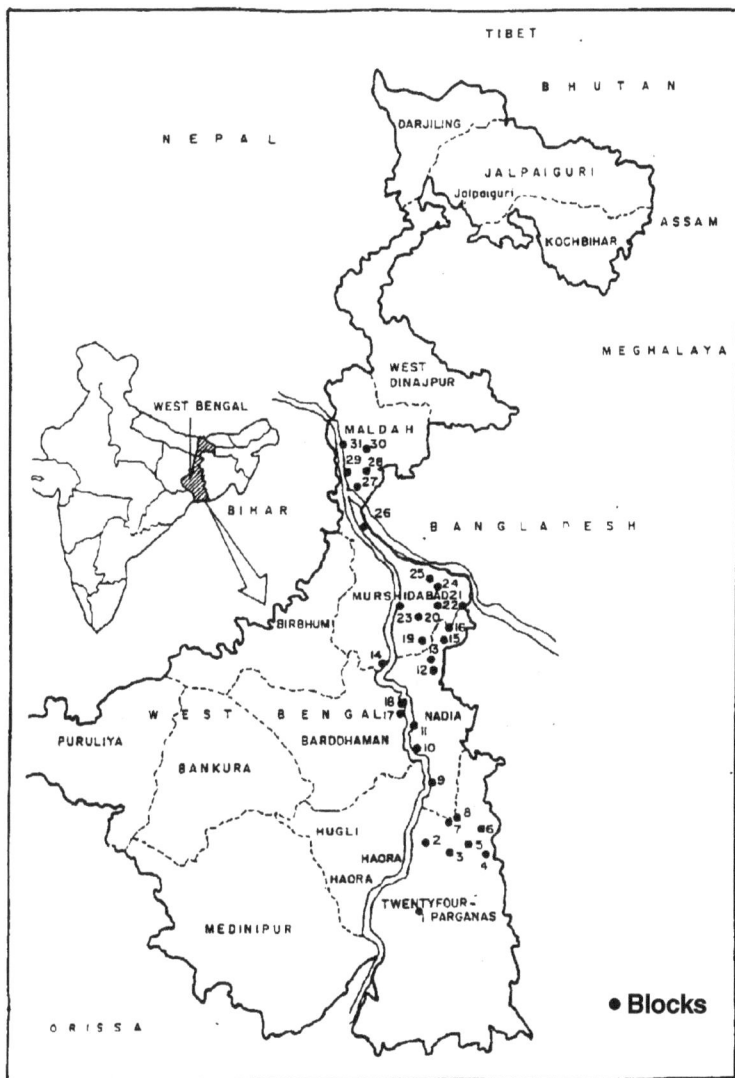

Figure III.1: Map Showing Arsenic Affected Six Districts

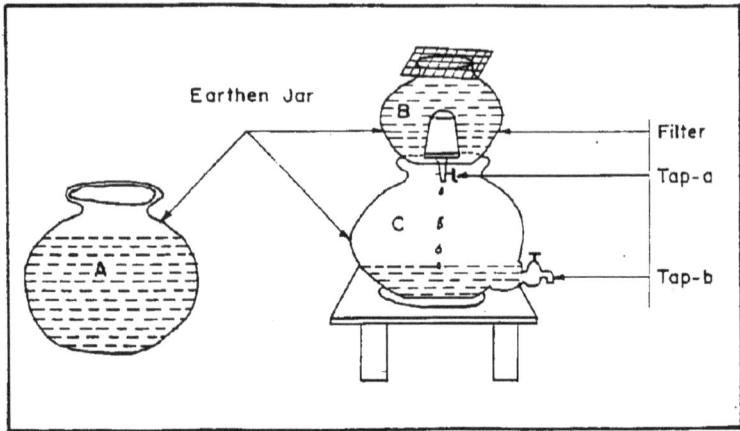

Figure III.2: Filtering System for Arsenic Removal

III.4 shows the diseases of the affected people of six districts (collaboration work with Dr. D.N. Guha Mazumder). Tables III.5 and III.6 show the results of some of the analyses of hair and urine.

The R and D work on arsenic has been taken up as a long term study by the SOES, Jadavpur University. One publication by Chakraborty *et al.*[117] mentions that the problem of arsenic in groundwater has now extended to seven districts of West Bengal. Their results indicate that the more the villages surveyed, the more arsenic affected areas and population are detected. Not only West Bengal, but the neighbouring country Bangladesh is also affected. The results of water analysis of Bangladesh conducted by SOES show that even in Narayanganj, Dhaka, which is far from arsenic affected areas of West Bengal, contains arsenic in groundwater upto 1.0 mg/L.

Table III.3: Arsenic Affected Districts in West Bengal

Districts in West Bengal and their names:

Koochbihar, Jalpaiguri, Darjeeling, West Dinajpur, Malda, Murshidabad, Nadia, Twentyfour Parganas (N), Twentyfour Parganas (S), Kolkata, Howrah, Hughli, Medinipur, Bankura, Purulia, Burdwan, Birbhum.

Affected districts in West Bengal and their names:

Malda, Murshidabad, Nadia, Twentyfour Parganas(North), Twentyfour Parganas(South), Burdwan.

* Area per cent of the affected districts compared to the total area of West Bengal: 38.47

* Population per cent of the affected districts compared to the total population of West Bengal: 44.4

Name of the block/police station of the six arsenic affected districts so far studied

Districts	Blocks
Malda	Kaliachalk-I, Kaliachalk-II, Kaliachalk-III, Englishbazar, Manikchalk
Murshidabad	Raninagar-I, Raninagar-II, Jalangi, Nawda, Hariharpara, Domkal, Baharampur, Suti-II
Nadia	Karimpur-I, Karimpur-II, Tehatta-I, Tehatta-II Nabwadip, Shantipur, Chakdaha, Kaliganj
Twentyfour Parganas (North)	Habra-1, Habra-II, Deganga, Baduria, Barasat, Swarupnagar, Basirhat**
Twentyfour Parganas (South)	Baruipur
Burdwan	Purbasthali-I, Purbasthali-II

*: This does not mean that total area and total population per cent are affected but the possibility cannot be ignored in long run.

**: Analysis was performed on 15.9.92, so we did not include its population and area.

Table III.4: Clinical Manifestation of Arsenic Poisoning

Initial stage: *Dermatitis, Karatitis, Conjunctivitis*, Rhinitis, Pharyngitis, Laryngitis, *Dronchitis, Gastroenteritis*.

Second stage: *Peripheral neuropathies*, Raynaud's Phenomenon, *Hepatopathy, Melanosis, Depigmentation, Hyperkeratosis*.

Late stage: Cardio and Cerebrovascular Disease, *Gangrene in the Limbs, Malignant Neoplasm*.

(*Italic* shows the manifestation observed among villagers).

Table III.5: Arsenic Levels in Hair Samples

Analyses of hair samples of the people showing arsenic manifestation in six districts of West Bengal

District	Range–ppm
Malda	4.93–11.13
Burdwan	6.92–7.24
Nadia	3.46–7.18
24(P) North and 24(P) South	4.6–12.5

*: Arsenic content in hair more than 2–3 ppm indicated possible poisoning.

*: Results of 1000 human hair was 0.5 ppm.

Table III.6: Arsenic Levels in Urine Samples

Urine arsenic level of the people drinking arsenic contaminated water in six districts of West Bengal, India

District	Range in µg/ml	Amount of Arsenic Excreted in Urine in µg per day (considering 1.5 litre* of urine for adult per day)
Murshidabad	0.143–1.286	214.5–1929
Nadia	0.286–1.429	429.0–2143.5
Malda Bardhaman	0.195–0.390	292.5–585
24 Parganas (South)	0.02–0.918	30.0–1377
24 Parganas (North)	0.163–1.00	244.5–1500

*: Per day arsenic excretion in urine should not be more than 5 µg.

*: *Principle of internal medicine*" by Harrison 12th edn., 1992. McGraw Hill Publication, p. 2182.

III.0.6 Organisation

National Geophysical Research Institute, Hyderabad.

Project Title

Geohydrological studies by NGRI in arsenic affected areas of West Bengal.

I. Natural Recharge Measurements

The NGRI has carried out natural recharge measurements to determine the quantum of annual replenishment of ground water, due to percolation of a fraction of the rainfall to the aquifers. This work was carried out in the 1995–96 hydrological cycle in different geological formations of the Arsenic affected North and South 24 Parganas districts and the Arsenic free Bankura district. The injected Tritium tracer technique was used. The results are:

(*i*) Bankura district

Formation	Natural Recharge
Granite gneiss	179 mm
Latterite	181 mm
Alluvium	137 mm

(*ii*) N 24 Parganas district

Alluvium (Rajarhat block)	198 mm

(*iii*) S 24 Parganas district

Alluvium (Baruipur and Sonarpur blocks)	34 mm

II. Work Proposed

(1) Water Harvesting and Artificial Recharge

Arsenic contamination of drinking water wells is a

recent phenomena, first noted about 20 years ago. The Arsenic affected area has increased in course of time and, at present, parts of seven districts are affected. The prevailing theory for recent manifestation of Arsenicosis proposes that excessive withdrawal of ground water leads to decline of water table, exposure to aeration of the dewatered clay beds containing Arsenopyrite and release of Arsenic from the clay beds to the ground water.

Taking into consideration the local hydrogeological situation, the NGRI has proposed the following pilot study to reduce the concentration of Arsenic in ground water.

The affected area has reasonably high seasonal rainfall (1500–2000 mm) and good ground water potential. The traditional method of Water Harvesting comprises construction of Pukurs (Village ponds). Every village has several such Pukurs. The surface water in the Pukurs is free from Arsenic. The NGRI has, therefore, proposed an Artificial Recharge experiment which will

(a) Improve the effective storage capacity of the water harvesting structure *i.e.* Pukur,

(b) Augment the local ground water reserve,

(c) Raise the water table level beneath the Pukur and thus reduce the thickness of the sub-surface layers exposed to oxidation and

(d) Dilute the Arsenic content of ground water.

The experiment comprises conversion of a Pukur into an infiltration basin and transfer of the Arsenic free surface water to the top aquifer directly or to the deeper confined aquifer through a tube well drilled at the bottom of the Pukur.

It is expected that a hand-pump located at a distance of 10–15 m from the experimental site will deliver water having Arsenic concentration below the permissible limit of 50 micrograms per litre.

The NGRI has carried out reconnaissance field surveys and has identified sites favourable for Artificial Recharge, (*i*) near Dattapukur, Barasat block, (*ii*) near Bininaypada, Habsa block, (*iii*) near Gobardonga, Gaighata block in N-24 Parganas district, and near Chakdah town, Chakdah block in Nadia district, for conducting the Artificial Recharge experiments.

(2) Dynamics of the Groundwater System

A better understanding of the genesis and spread of Arsenic contamination of the ground water can develop only after measurement of the aquifer parameters such as storage coefficient and transmissivity and the physical juxtaposition of the intercalating sand/clay layers. The NGRI proposes to undertake these measurements in two selected watersheds.

Information on the dynamics o£ the ground water system in terms of its age, residence time, velocity and interconnection with surface water bodies is needed. Isotope hydrological studies involving measurement of Tritium, Radiocarbon, Deuterium and Oxygen-18 are required for eliciting this information. NGRI has initiated studies on this aspect in collaboration with the Isotope group of Bhabha Atomic Research Centre, Mumbai.

(3) Pattern of Arsenic Distribution

NGRI has prepared a heirarchial stratigraphic sampling scheme for periodic collection of ground water samples from 750 wells, tapping aquifers at three different depths and located in both the affected and unaffected areas of six districts.

Annexure IV

Groundwater Development in the Arsenic-Affected Alluvial Belt of West Bengal: Some Questions

Hydrogeology

It is now recognized that a huge alluvial tract bound by the Bhagirathi (Ganga) river in the West. Malda district in the North and 24-Parganas in the South (eastern boundary perhaps extending into Bangladesh territory) is affected by arsenic pollution of groundwater. The western part of Bengal, *i.e.* west of Bhagirathi river is not reported to have been hit. Also the northern part or the sub-

Himalayan areas of West Bengal *i.e.* West Dinajpur and Coochbehar districts, are as yet unaffected. Is Nature angry with the people of the eastern belt? What is the significance of this selective contamination from the hydrogeological point of view (Figure IV.1).

The Bengal basin has four phases of depositions and erosions coinciding with four inter-glacial and glacial periods in the Quaternary lime (0 to 1.6 million/years). Prior to the recent deposition of Sunderban Delta and active river banks, a deposition took place some time between 25,000 and 80,000 years ago (commonly known as the younger deltaic deposits, YDD). The sediments were mainly brought by the Ganga (Belt I in Figure IV.1).

The major part of the western alluvial belt (Belt II in Figure IV.1) called the Older Deltaic Plain (ODP) developed during Quaternary time between 80.000 and 1.6 million years ago by 2 or 3 glacial-interglacial cycles with sea level fall and rise coinciding with the glacial and de-glaciation phases respectively. Sea level fall (*i.e.* Bay of Bengal's fall) results in an erosional phase and sea level rise results in depositional aspects in the river system. These sediments were brought from the Chotanagpur plateau of Bihar by easterly flowing river systems like the Ajay-Damodar-Subarnarekha.

ODP extends into the sub-surface below the arsenic belt (YDP) and takes its proper stratigraphic position. That is why perhaps deeper aquifers under the arsenic belt are as yet free from arsenic contamination.

The sediments comprising most part of the districts of West Dinajpur, Coochbehar etc. (Belt III in Figure IV.1) were

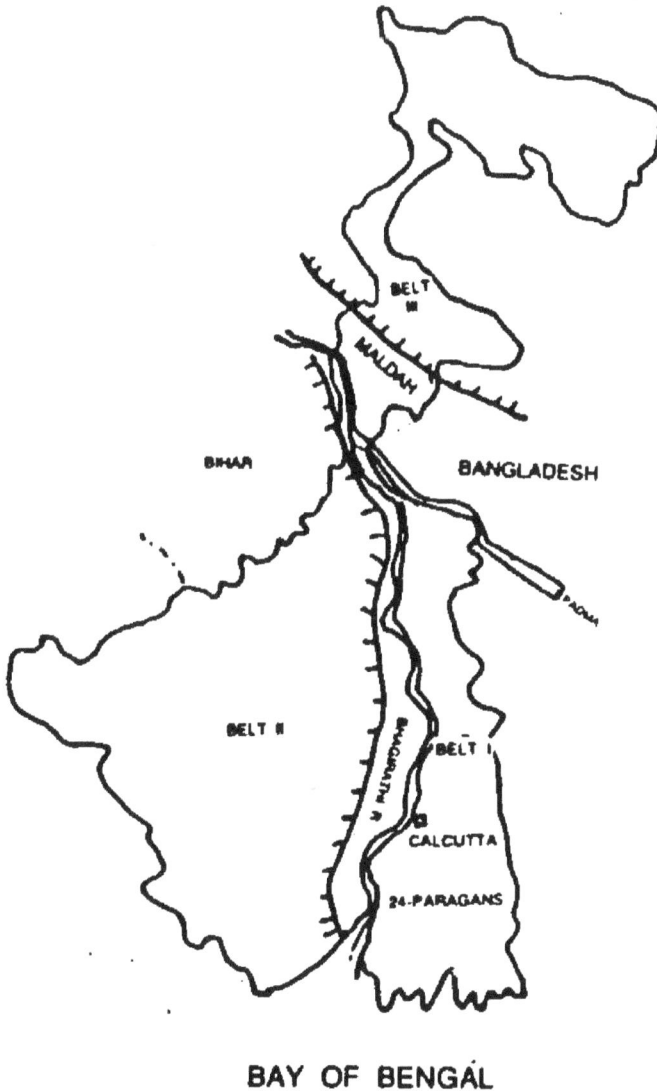

BAY OF BENGÁL

Figure IV.1: Map Showing Three Broad Divisions with respect
to Occurrence/Absence of Arsenic in Groundwater.
Belt 1 is the arsenic-affected division consisting of
sediments brought by the Ganga; Belts II and III are
arsenic-free zones consisting of sediments brought
by rivers other than the Ganga.

brought by Himalayan river coming from the North and therefore are different from the Ganga sediments.

Groundwater Development Structures

It is known that billions of litres of water have been and are being pumped out every year from this belt with the help of groundwater structures (Table IV.1).

Working Schedule

Except during the rainy season (June to September), irrigation pumps are run for a few hours almost daily to irrigate the nearby fields. Pumping for eight hours per day is common. It has been estimated that on the average an irrigation pump runs for about 500–800 hours a year. Water supply tubewells, however, run throughout the year.

Arsenic Mixing in the Aquifers

In our earlier model we attempted to show how there was increased supply of oxygen to groundwater[2]. The cause of this increased supply of oxygen is due to the operation of tubewells known to cause extension of vadose zones (VZ). *i.e.* unsaturated air-water mixed zones (Zs) (Figure IV.2), during pumping, thereby supplying more oxygen/ dissolved air with oxygen as an important constituent to the groundwater.

It is, therefore, expected that though arsenic-bearing bed (layer) may be found throughout the five districts (in the eastern belt) in discontinuous forms (lenses), the release of arsenic will take place only around the areas (VZs and Zs) where increased supply of oxygen/dissolved air is available and is reacting with the arsenic-bearing formation. It is to be noted that the arsenic-bearing deposits can neither occur at a uniform depth nor can have uniform thickness.

Table IV.1: Groundwater Structures Operating in the Arsenic-Affected Alluvial Belt of West Bengal

Specifications	Heavy/Medium Duty Tubewells	Shallow (Low duty) Tubewells	Tubewell with Hand Pump
Depth range	50 to 200m	30 to 100m	10 to 200m
Tapping zone(s) thickness (average)	30m	10m	3–5 m
Size and design	(35 cm × 20 cm) (14" × 8") or (30 cm × 15cm) (12" × 6") or (20 cm × 10cm) (8" × 4") diameter	(7 cm or 10 cm) (3" or 4") diameter	(5 cm to 10 cm) (2" to 4") diameter
Drawdown	6 to 12m	3 to 6m	Insignificant
Discharge	100 m³/h	20 m³/h	Small, discontinuous
Borehole	Gravel packed	Gravel/cause sand packed	No specification
Use	Irrigation/water supply	Irrigation/water supply	Domestic water supply
Numbers	About 3000	About 1 lakh	Over 5 lakh
Pump	Electric/diesel pump > 10 HP	Electric/diesel pump ≥ 5 HP	Hand pump

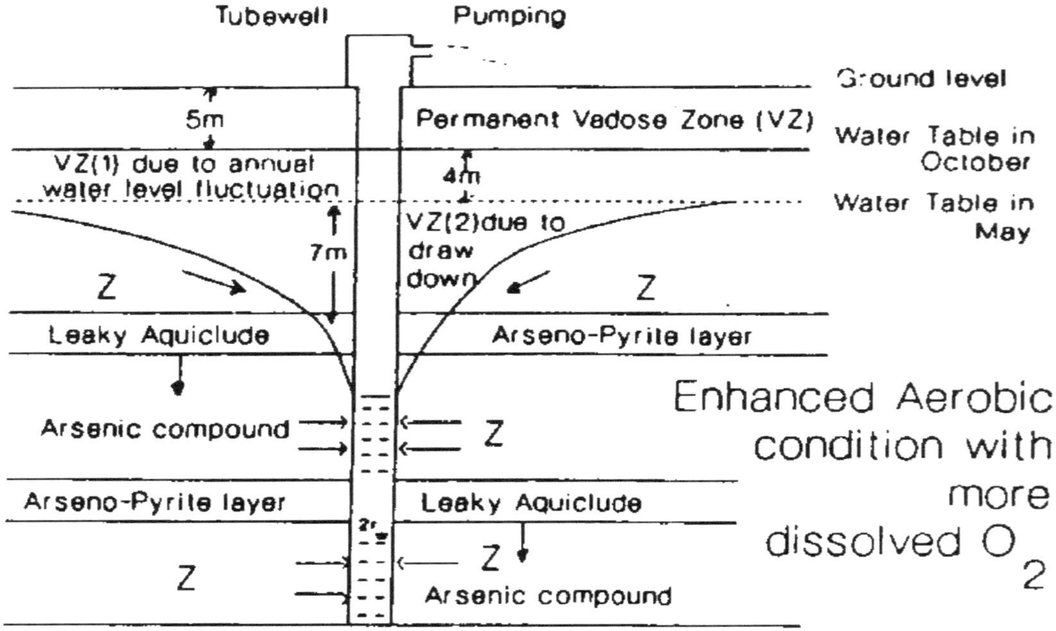

Figure IV.2: Aerobic Condition in Groundwater Around a Heavy Duty Tubewell in the Eastern Part of West Bengal. VZ(1) and VZ(2) are dynamic vadose zones, these and Zs are the mixing zones due to tubewell pumping.

In normal conditions groundwater movement (velocity) is very slow in the arsenic-affected tract of West Bengal owing to its flat nature (average slope is 10 cm/km). The groundwater movement is of the order of 500 cm per year in horizontal direction and still less as far as vertical movement is concerned. Vertical movement, however, is much faster in the vadose zone (VZ in Figure IV.2) created by annual water level fluctuation (about 4 m in VZ(1), rectangular and wide spread) and due to draw down, during pumping [up to 10m in VZ(2) in an inverted conical form Figure IV.2). What happens daily is a downward movement of water-air particles in VZ(2) zone during pumping and upward movement when the pump is slopped after a few hours.

Leaving aside this mixing mechanism. one may examine the velocity of groundwater in the vicinity of the strainer (or slotted pipe) of the tubewell deep under ground in the aquifer, when the pump is in operation (in zone Z in Figure N.2). If Q is the steady state discharge of a tubewell pumping water continuously then the same Q amount of water must enter the tubewell through the strainer pores to maintain the discharge.

Therefore,

Q = Velocity (V) × Pore area of the strainer (A)

A = x% of $2\pi r_w h$, where r_w = radius of the strainer. h = length of strainer and x% is the percentage of open space in the strainer which in field conditions varies from 30 to 70 per cent.

For heavy/medium duty tubewells and shallow tubewells the value of V varies from 0.01 to 05 cm/sec. This is several thousand times more than the convective velocity of natural groundwater (or groundwater in unexploited aquifer).

What is the velocity, a few meters away from the strainer?

Normally a velocity gradient is created around the tubewell strainer and spreads at least up to the limit of the cone of depression. This value is of the order of 250 m radius in case of heavy duty tubewell and 50m in case of shallow tubewells. Velocity is maximum at the entrance points where $r = r_w$ and minimum (tending to zero) at the outer surface of the cylinder of influence having equivalent radius of the cone of depression.

In other words, each tubewell while in operation is acting as a stirrer (a spoon in a tea cup) for an aquifer of cylindrical volume of about 50 to 250 m radius with its height being the entire depth of the tubewell strainer (Zs in Figure N.2). If the source of arsenic is located somewhere in this zone, it can get mixed up with the entire volume of the tubewell's effective influence zone within a short time. Otherwise, perhaps it would have taken thousands of years for the arsenic to spread in the natural course, through dispersion-convection mechanism.

Consider a situation where thousands and thousands of tubewell are running in the arsenic-affected alluvial belt simultaneously. The predominant parameter for mixing will depend on a convection-dispersion model in which convective velocity will be overwhelming compared to dispersion. Thus the pollutant's scattering by spreading around the mean flow (dispersion) will be far less contributing to the overall spread (mixing) than the pollutant's physical movement with the mean flow (convection).

Phenomena Contributing to Mitigation

Keeping in mind that a large area (several thousand square kilometers) of aquifer has been affected and that it is not possible to stop the spreading of underground arsenic once the process of leaching has been triggered, let us examine what are the factors which contribute to the alleviation of arsenic pollution.

(*i*) Recharge of arsenic-free rainwater. It is an established fact that every year about 4 m of aquifer water column, on the average, is getting recharged at the top of the summer (lowest) water table. This is equivalent to about 50cm of rainwater amounting to half a million m^3 of water per sq km area. This huge amount of water is arsenic-free. If we can get this recharged water mixed with the shallow aquifer, say within 50m of depth and also withdraw this water annually, then mitigation is started. For this purpose, future tubewells of all duty can be restricted to a depth of 50 m. so that these act as underground mixing tools as well as tubewells for the purposes that they are being used now.

(*ii*) The arsenic removal system patented by CSIR-Jadavpur University could be used more pervasively in the areas where arsenic contamination in groundwater is observed.

(*iii*) It is not advisable to exploit deeper aquifers extensively as they may ultimately get contaminated with arsenic. The safe limit of arsenic in drinking water is so low (0.02 ppm) and the mixing phenomenon by tubewells is so prominent that exploitation of underlying deeper aquifer may not be feasible without running the risk of it getting contaminated after some time. Also, mitigating deeper aquifer is more difficult and costlier than manipulating/managing the shallow aquifers.

In conclusion, it is reiterated that all the above discussions are based on the fact that the source of arsenic is geological and the mixing mechanism originates from arsenic-leaching. This has to be established by further scientific work. An idea about the occurrence of arsenic-bearing layers and the amount that can be leached out to the aquifer under present conditions are to be investigated. A mathematical modelling approach backed by borehole data may perhaps form the basis of such studies.

References

1. Mallick, S. and Niyogi. D., *Indian Geohydrol.*, 1972, 8: 86–99.

2. Mallick, S. and Rajagopal, N.R., *J. Sci. Ind. Res.*, 1995, 54: 329–330.

3. Saha, A K. Annual Volume, 1991, Centre for Study of Man and Environment. Presidency College. Calcutta.

Annexure V
Treatability Studies Conducted by NEERI

V.1 Coagulation-flocculation

Water treatment with metal coagulants like alum and ferric chloride has long been recognized as an effective method for the removal of arsenic. NEERI conducted coagulation-flocculation studies on arsenic removal on water samples collected from six sources in West Bengal which are affected by arsenic. The physico-chemical characteristics of these water samples are given in Tables V.I and V.2. Extensive treatability studies have shown that a dose of 3.0 mg/L of chlorine (for prechlorination) followed by 50 mg/L of ferric chloride was able to bring down the arsenic level in treated water below 25 µg/L from the worst affected samples. The results are presented in Table V.3.

Table V.I: Levels of Arsenic, Iron and Manganese in Groundwaters of West Bengal

Sample No.	Location	Source	Depth in m	Concentration (mg/L)		
				As	Fe	Mn
IA	Kalsur	Handpump (Private)	15.85	0.89	4.43	0.27
IIA	Bishnupur	Handpump (Private)	21.33	0.64	4.44	1.13
IIIA	Ramnagar	Handpump (Private)	30.48	0.61	4.42	0.97
IB	Chandalhati	Handpump (PHED)	140.21	0.06	3.00	0.29
IIB	Bishnupur	Handpump (PHED)	14.02	0.01	0.65	0.05
IIIB	Piyali	Handpump (PHED)	304.80	0.01	0.22	0.17

Table V.2: Physico-Chemical Characteristics of Groundwater Samples of West Bengal (Date of Sampling : April 18, 1996)

Sl.No.	Parameter	Sampling Points (Depth)					
		IA (15.85m)	IIA (21.36m)	IIIA (30.48 m)	IB (140.21m)	IIB (14.02m)	IIIB (304.8 m)
1.	pH	7.3	7.3	7.3	7.3	7.7	7.6
2.	Conductivity (µS/cm)	768	730	710	800	785	860
3.	Total-Alkalinity (mg/L, $CaCO_3$)	392	378	372	428	398	392
4.	Total Hardness (mg/L, $CaCO_3$)	356	360	348	390	320	264
5.	Calcium (mg/L, Ca)	97	103	100	112	92	62
6.	Magnesium (mg/L, Mg)	28	25	24	27	22	26
7.	Chlorides (mg/L, Cl)	26	18	18	16	28	38
8.	Sulphates (mg/L, SO_4)	ND	ND	ND	ND	1	31
9.	Nitrates (mg/L, N)	0.3	0.4	0.4	0.3	0.3	ND
10.	Sodium (mg/L, Na)	36	26	27	36	65	125
11.	Potassium (mg/L, K)	3	3	3	4	3	4
12.	Arsenic* (mg/L, As)	0.89	.64	0.61	0.06	0.01	0.01

ND: Not Detectable.

*: Permissible limit for Arsenic: 0.05 mg/L as per BIS and WHO Standards.

Table V.3: Arsenic Removal Studies on Groundwaters of West Bengal

Sample No.	Location/District	Chlorine mg/L	Ferric Chloride mg/L	pH	Cond. µS/cm	Total Alkalinity mg/L as CaCo₃	Arsenic* mg/L R.W.	Arsenic* mg/L T.W.	Removal %
IA	Handpump at Kalsur 24 Parganas (North)	0	0	7.3	768	392	0.740	–	–
		0	50	7.6	746	328	–	0.037	95.0
		3.0	50	74	846	356	–	ND	100.0
IIA	Handpump at Bishnupur 24 Parganas (North)	0	0	7.3	730	378	0.510	–	–
		0	50	7.7	780	314	–	0.037	92.7
		3.0	50	7.4	802	344	>	0.002	99.6
IIIA	Handpump at Ramnagar 24 Parganas (South)	0	0	7.3	710	372	0.490	–	–
		0	50	7.6	723	318	–	0.100	79.6
		3.0	50	7.3	778	324	–	0.14	97.1
IB	Handpump at Chandalhati 24 Parganas (North)	0	0	7.3	800	428	0.014	–	–
		3.0	30	7.5	828	402	–	ND	100.0

Contd...

Table V.3–Contd...

Sample No.	Location/District	Chlorine mg/L	Ferric Chloride mg/L	pH	Cond. µS/cm	Total Alkalinity mg/L as CaCo₃	Arsenic* mg/L R.W.	Arsenic* mg/L T.W	Removal %
IIB	Handpump at Bishnupur 24 Parganas (North)	0 3.0	0 30	7.7 7.6	785 702	398 365	0.014 –	– ND	– 100 0
IIIB	Handpump at Piyali 24 Parganas (South)	0 3.0	0 30	7.6 7	860 886	392 360	ND –	– ND	– 100.0

RW: Raw Water; TW: Treated Water; ND: Not detetable.

* Permissible limit for Arsenic: 0.05 mg/L as per BIS and WHO Standards.

Table V.4: Arsenic Removal from West Bengal Samples (Adsorption Studies with Bauxite)

Volume of material in column–100 mL; Particle Size: 0.8–1.4 mm; Feed water flow: 10 mL/min

Sl.No.	Sample No.	Location/District	Feed Water As µg/L	Treated Water Arsenic µg/L					
				NALCO				Phutakapar (BALCO)	
				Heat Treated		Acid and Heat Treated		Heat Treated	
				A	B	A	B	A	B
1.	IA	Hand Pump at Kalsur 24 Paraganas (North)	906	8.2	10.2	8.5	10.9	7.7	9.8
2.	IIA	Hand Pump at Bishnupur 24 Paraganas (North)	349	9.1	11.6	7.6	9.7	6.3	7.3
3.	IIIA	Hand Pump at Ramnagar 24 Paraganas (South)	361	6.4	10.0	4.6	5.9	6.8	9.6

A: Composite sample of 5 bed volume; B: Grab sample after 5 bed volume;
Permissible limit for arsenic: 0.05 mg/L as per BIS and WHO standards.

V.2 Adsorption

Adsorption studies conducted by NEERI on samples of bauxite procured from the Jawaharlal Nehru Aluminium Research Centre, Nagpur were found to bring down the arsenic level in the groundwater samples of West Bengal to below 25 µg/L. The results of these probing studies are at Table V.4.

Annexure VI
Studies on Arsenic Contamination in Drinking Water by AIIH&PH, Kolkata

List of Research Studies on Arsenic Contamination in Drinking water undertaken by All India Institute of Hygiene and Public Health, Kolkata

1. Study on Chronic Arsenic Toxicity from drinking tubewell water in rural West Bengal. 'Conducted by All India Institute of Hygiene and Public Health and School of Tropical Medicine, 1985 to 1987.

2. Study on Arsenic Pollution in Ground Water in West Bengal–A submission Project of National Drinking Water Mission. Study conducted by All

India Institute of Hygiene and Public Health (AIIH&PH). School of Tropical Medicine (STM), Centre for Studies of Man and Environment (CSME), State Water Investigation Directorate (SWID), Central Ground Water Board (CGWB) and Public Health Engineering Directorate (PHED), Government of West Bengal, 1988-91.

3. Development of Appropriate Field Method for Removal of Arsenic from Ground Water (Res. Project sponsored by National Drinking Water Mission (NDWM), Ministry of Rural Areas and Employment (MRAE), Government of India. Study conducted by AIIH&PH, 1991–93.

4. Arsenic Pollution in Ground Water in West Bengal. Investigation by the Committee constituted by Government of West Bengal vide notification No. PHE-I/716/3D-1/88 Part-1 dated the 6th April, 1992. Investigation conducted by All India Institute of Hygiene and Public Health (AIIH&PH), Central Ground Water Board (CGWB), Centre for Studies of Man and Environment (CSME), State Water Investigation Directorate (SWID), School of Tropical Medicine (STM), Public Health Engineering Directorate (PHED), (Government of West Bengal). Jadavpur University, Bardhaman University, 1992-94.

5. Development of Field Testing Kit for Arsenic Estimation (sponsored by UNICEF). Study undertaken by AIIH&PH during 1995–97.

6. Epidemiological, Clinical and Therapeutical study in Arsenic affected districts of West Bengal

(sponsored by Ministry of Health and Family Welfare, Government of West Bengal). Study undertaken by AIIH&PH (1996).

7. Study on Chronic Arsenic Toxicity to assess total extent and magnitude of the impact of Arsenic contamination in ground water in West Bengal (sponsored by Ministry of Health and Family Welfare, Government of India). Conducted by AIIH&PH.

8. Comprehensive Capacity Building, Training and Awareness Generation Programme to tackle the arsenic problem in West Bengal. Conducted by AIIH&PH in collaboration with World Health Organisation, PHED, Government of West Bengal (1997).

Arsenic in Ground Water: Methodology for Removal (Year 1997)

Prof. K.J. Nath[1] and Prof. A. Majumder[2]

1.0 Introduction

In nature Arsenic is widely distributed. Though arsenic has served mankind well in different ways, it is often viewed as being synonymous with toxic. The sources of arsenic in soil are mainly the parent (or rock) materials from which it is derived. The most important ores of arsenic are arsenic pyrites or mispickel (FeAsS), realgar (As_4S_4) and orpiment (As_2S_3).

In West Bengal arsenic contamination in ground water has been reported mainly from six districts (Malda, Murshidabad, Nadia, North 24-Parganas, South 24-

1 Director, All India Institute of Hygiene and Public Health, Kolkata, India.

2 Professor of Environmental Sanitation, Department of Sanitary Engineering, All India Institute of Hygiene and Public Health, 110, Chittaranjan Avenue, Kolkata – 700 073, India.

Parganas and Bardhaman). The arsenic affected area is a part of the Ganga-Brahmaputra delta having a near surface succession of Quarternary Sediments of varying thickness. The reported occurrences of arsenic above permissible limit are all confined within meander belt zone of the upper delta plain comprising Late Quarternary Sediments.

In rural areas/ground water is supplied mostly because treatment including disinfection is often not required. Hand pumps to draw ground water are placed near the consumers for direct use. If arsenic is present in ground water then it can be removed by several methods. If ground water with arsenic are treated through oxidation, sedimentation and filtration steps for removal of iron and manganese, simultaneously arsenic concentration goes down considerably. Thus the removed arsenic, since bound in sludge, pose problem for disposal of the residue.

In the above context, it would be appropriate to explore thoroughly all the possible methods of removal of arsenic from drinking water and to arrive at appropriate technology which could be used for upgradation of water quality in arsenic affected areas of West Bengal.

2.0 Treatment Options

The following methods could be used for removal of arsenic from drinking water:

(*i*) Oxidation of Arsenic (III)

(*ii*) Coagulation-flocculation-sedimentation-filtration

(*iii*) Ion exchange

(*iv*) Adsorption

(*v*) Osmosis or electrodialysis.

The effective removal of arsenic from water requires complete oxidation of Arsenic (III). There are several chemical oxidants available for such oxidation. However, considering it to be used for drinking water treatment, selection of oxidant is very important.

Conventional coagulation flocculation and filtration may be used for removal of Arsenic. Cadmium, Chromium, Copper, Lead, Selenium, Silver etc. pH adjustment is considered to be an important factor in effective removal operation. Arsenic, Barium, Cadmium, Chromium, Fluoride, Lead, Silver, etc. may also be removed from water by the application of excess lime. However, in such case pH in water will stand around 11.0.

Table VI.1: Treatment Options for Contaminants Removal

Sl.No.	Treatment Options	Contaminants Removed
1.	Coagulation-flocculation-Sedimentation-filtration	Arsenic, Cadmium, Chromium, Copper, Lead. Selenium, Silver etc.
2.	Excess lime treatment	Arsenic, Barium, Cadmium, Chromium, Fluoride, Lead, Silver, etc.
3.	Activated alumina or Activated granular carbon	Arsenic, Fluoride, Selenium, etc.
4.	Ion Exchange	Arsenic, Barium, Cadmium, Chromium, Copper, Lead, Nitrate etc.
5.	Reverse Osmosis	Arsenic, Barium, Cadmium, Chromium, Copper, Fluoride, Lead, Nitrate, Silver etc.

Arsenic, Fluoride, Selenium etc. could be removed by the principle of adsorption through activated alumina or granular carbon. Ion exchange has been found to be effective in removing Arsenic, Barium, Cadmium, Chromium, Copper, Lead, Nitrate, etc. from drinking water. Reverse osmosis method could be used for removal of Arsenic, Barium, Cadmium Chromium, Copper, Fluoride, Lead, Nitrate, Selenium, Silver etc. also. However, if some inorganics could be present as suspended solids in water then to remove these direct filtration technique may be adopted. Table VI.1 highlights the various treatment options for removal of certain inorganics.

3.0 Methodology

Arsenic occurs in aquatic environment in trivalent (Arsenite) or pentavalent (Arsenate) form and these forms are considered to be most important in selecting removal methodology. It was reported that as a general rule, arsenite is more likely to be found in anaerobic ground water and arsenate in aerobic surface water. In geogenic arsenic the two valence forms of arsenic (Arsenite and Arsenate) are probably the only species of concern. The chemical behaviour of the two forms are different and as such during removal of arsenic, concentration of each redox species need to be estimated. Different studies indicate that Arsenic (III) cannot be removed from water effectively. Hence, during removal process arsenite may preferably be oxidised to arsenate. There are several methods available which could be used for removal of arsenic from drinking water. These methods are as follows:

- (*i*) Oxidation of Arsenic (III)
- (*ii*) Coagulation-flocculation-Sedimentation-filtration (Co-Precipitation)
- (*iii*) Ion exchange

(*iv*) Adsorption

(*v*) Osmosis or electrodialysis

4.0 Case Study

All India Institute of Hygiene and Public Health carried out R&D studies on removal of arsenic from drinking water. Both laboratory and field scale pilot studies were carried out by the application of different methodologies. The findings of different studies are briefly presented below:

4.1 Oxidation-Coagulation Flocculation-Sedimentation (Co-precipitation Technique)

Oxidation of As (III) by dissolved oxygen in water is a very slow process. In oxygen free ground water, a part of arsenic may be present in arsenite form. But effective removal of arsenic from water requires complete oxidation of As(III). Accordingly selection of appropriate oxidising agent is a very important task. The following criteria are required to be considered for selection of appropriate oxidising agent:

(*i*) Residual effect

(*ii*) Oxidation by-products

(*iii*) Oxidation of other inorganic and organic water constituents

(*iv*) Reaction kinetics.

On the basis of availability of oxidants it is considered that bleaching powder solution would be most appropriate for oxidising As (III) to As (V) during removal. As there remains some residual effect of chlorine in water, it is recommended that dosage of chlorine must be restricted within 0.5 mg/L. Such a dose would also restrict the residual effect of chlorine to less than 0.2 mg/L in the treated water. Moreover chlorine dose would take care of bacteriological contamination, if any, during the water treatment process.

The next step of co-precipitation process is coagulation-flocculation. The common use of aluminium and ferric salts in drinking water treatment is primarily for coagulation of particles and colloids in the water. Both metal salts undergo hydrolysis to various products, but can be reduced to a very low residual if the poorly soluble hydroxides are formed at the proper pH and can be filtered off completely. Dissolved substances, such as heavy metals, phosphates and humic substances, can also be bound to the precipitate by adsorption or they may even precipitates directly. Field as well as laboratory studies carried out by AIIH&PH indicated that alum salt or ferric salt in the tune of 30–60 mg/L or 20–40 mg/L respectively could be added for coagulation. The addition rapid mixing for 60 seconds followed by very slow mixing for a couple of minutes for development of flocs must be carried out. Such flocs are then allowed to be settled at the bottom. The settling time requirement is generally not less than 30 minutes (Preferably 1 hr.).

The supernatant water is then required to be filtered through selected filtering media. The filtering media used during the study was domestic candle, gravel and sand-gravel.

The efficacy of different coagulants were tested both in laboratory and field and the following results were obtained (Table VI.2). Initially, bleaching powder amounting to 2 mg/L was added to convert Arsenic (III) to Arsenic (V). The water was filtered after co-precipitation.

Table VI.2: Different Coagulants Tested for Arsenic Removal

Location of Groundwater	Arsenic Content (as As mg/L) in Raw Water	Added Chemical	Arsenic content in Treated Water (mg/L)	pH
Katchua, Habra-II North 24–Parganas	0.26	Ferrous Sulphate	0.13	8.0
–do–	0.26	Ferric Chloride	0.03	9.0
–do–	0.26	Aluminium Sulphate	0.02	7.5
–do–	0.26	Lime	0.19	11.0
Dattapukur, Barasat, North 24–Parganas	0.15	Ferrous Sulphate	0.09	8.2
–do–	0.15	Ferric Chloride	0.02	8.7
–do–	0.15	Aluminium Sulphate	0.01	7.4
–do–	0.15	Lime	0.01	10.6

Performance of alum in removal of Arsenic as co-precipitation was monitored for different samples of water. One of the test results for removal of Arsenic from ground water containing 0.335 mg/L of Arsenic are presented in Table VI.3.

Table VI.3: Effect of Alum Dosage on Arsenic Removal

Dosage of Alum (mg/L)	Control pH by Adding Lime	Conc. of Arsenic after Treatment	Per cent of Removal Arsenic
10	7.5	0.11	67.16
20	7.3	0.07	79.10
30	7.2	0.05	85.07
40	7.2	0.03	91.04
50	7.3	0.02	94.02
60	7.2	0.01	97.00

Initial Concentration of Arsenic in Raw (Ground) Water = 0.3353 mg/L; Initial pH = 7.1; B.P. added : 2 mg/L.

The performance indicates that rate of removal of Arsenic is dependent on remaining concentration of Arsenic in water. The curve also indicates higher percentage of removal of Arsenic from water at higher Alum dose. However, an optional dose could be derived for removal of Arsenic and it is dependent on initial concentration of arsenic in ground water. The pH control is necessary during the process of co-precipitation. Generally pH in the range between 7 and 8 is considered to be ideal. Laboratory study also indicated that when pH of the water went below 7, the removal of arsenic at optimum dose of Aluminium sulphate was unsatisfactory. By adding 60 mg/L of alum satisfactory removal of arsenic was achieved.

The performance of addition of ferrous sulphate for removal of arsenic was also monitored in laboratory (Table VI.4). Initially bleaching powder was added to convert arsenite to arsenate, if any, in the raw water.

Table VI.4: Effect of Ferrous Sulphate Dosage on Arsenic Removal

Raw Water Arsenic Content (mg/L)	B.P. as Chlorine Dose (mg/L)	Ferrous Sulphate (mg/L)	Lime (CaO) (mg/L)	Arsenic Content after Treatment	Per cent Removal
0.21	0.5	10	2	0.14	35
0.21	0.5	20	4	0.06	75
0.21	0.5	40	8	0.03	86
0.21	0.5	80	16	0.01	95
0.21	0.5	120	24	Nil	100

In all the methodologies described above, flash and slow mixing after addition of coagulants are important. A minimum detention time of 30 minutes prior to filtration is found to be essential. However one hour detention prior to filtration would be ideal for the purpose.

A significant removal of arsenic was noticed at lesser dose of coagulant when iron content in ground water was more than 1 mg/L. Both sand filtration technique and candle filtration technique were used in the laboratory for final removal of precipitation of arsenic in water.

The laboratory study indicated that if prolonged settling (more than 12 hours) could be provided then arsenic removal in the tune of 65 per cent to 85 per cent could be achieved. Table VI.5 highlight the removal of arsenic by the process of oxidation (B.P. addition), coagulation-flocculation (alum addition) and settling.

**Table VI.5: Arsenic Removal by Oxidation, Coagulation-
Flocculation and Settling**

Initial Arsenic in Drinking Water	Arsenic Content in Drinking Water after Treatment but without Filtration	Efficiency
0.16	0.05	68 per cent
0.27	0.03	88 per cent
0.26	0.07	73 per cent

4.1.2 Application of Co-precipitation Method

4.1.2.1 Domestic Filter

Domestic filters have been developed by AIIH&PH with candle filters as well as sand-gravel filter. Domestic filter fitted with two-candle filters can produce 30 liters per day arsenic free water. Similarly sand-gravel G.I. domestic-filter (30 cm × 25 cm × 35 cm) can produce 300 liters/day arsenic free water.

Both types of above mentioned domestic filters have been tested in the field by the Central Ground Water Board. The performance during field trial was found to be satisfactory. A few such filters have been supplied to the Public Health Engineering Directorate, Government of West Bengal for Performance evaluation. The salient features of the domestic filter are presented in Table VI.6.

4.1.2.2 Arsenic Removal Plant with Piped Water Supply Schemes

In 1993 AIIH&PH carried out field experiment for removal of Arsenic in collaboration with the Executive Engineer, Malda Division, P.H. Engineering Directorate for Jatgopal-Kagmari Water Supply Scheme. The existing iron removal plant for the W/S scheme was utilised for Arsenic

Table VI.6: Salient Features of Domestic Filter (Year 1997)

☆ Cost of candle filters fitted with plastic bucket	Rs. 250/-
☆ Cost of G.I. Sand Gravel filter	Rs. 450/-
☆ Cleaning intervals of filter	15 days
☆ Life of candle filter	1 year
☆ Cost of each candle filter	Rs. 35/-
☆ Running cost of candle filter	10 p./day
☆ Running cost of G.I. sand gravel filter	20 p./day

removal. Alum salt was used as the coagulant. Field study showed encouraging result of arsenic removal by Creating 36000 lt/day water. The P.H. Engineering Department has already installed an Arsenic Removal Plant attached to piped W/S scheme at Sujapur, Malda. It is reported that the plant is running satisfactorily.

4.1.2.3 Handpump Attached Arsenic Removal Plant

AIIH&PH has developed a model of Hand-Pump attached Arsenic Removal Plant (HP-ARP). The unit has been installed in collaboration with 'Save the Environment', an NGO at Asokenagar. The principle of functioning of the ARP is oxidation-coagulation-flocculation-sedimentation-filtration (oxicoflocsedfil). The plant has been designed on the basis of maximum treatment rate of 1000 litres/hour. The raw water contains 0.19 mg/L of Arsenic and 2.8 mg/L of iron. The Arsenic and iron in filtered water have been found to be 0.005 mg/L and 0.18 mg/L respectively (Table VI.7).

The performance of Arsenic removal by co-precipitation in handpump attached arsenic removal plant showed that since iron content in the raw water was 2.8 mg/L and as adequate oxidation of iron was taken place in the ARP

Table VI.7: Performance (Trial Run) of Handpump Attached Arsenic Removal Plant (November–December, 1996)

Raw (TW) Water Quality		Chlorine Dosage (mg/L)	Alum Dosage (mg/L)	Rate of Treatment (lt/hr.)	Treated Water Quality	
Arsenic (mg/L)	Iron (mg/L)				Iron (mg/L)	Arsenic (mg/L)
0.19	2.8	Nil	Nil	525	0.72	0.06
0.19	2.8	Nil	Nil	525	0.69	0.055
0.19	2.8	0.5	25	525	0.36	0.025
0.19	2.8	0.5	30	525	0.34	0.02
0.19	2.8	0.5	40	525	0.20	0.005
0.19	2.8	0.5	40	525	0.18	BDL
0.19	2.8	0.5	40	525	0.18	0.005

considerable quantum of arsenic (arsenate) came out as co-precipitate of iron floe. However, with the increase of alum dosage residual arsenic decreased satisfactorily. It was found that 40 mg/L of alum dose would be the optimum dosage of coagulant.

Salient Information on HP-ARP

Rate of filtration (max.)	1000 litre/hr.
Mixing zone	Baffle type
Flocculation zone	Circular
Sedimentation zone	Circular
Filtration system	Upflow
Filter media	Gravel (3 to 5 mm)
Filtration rate	1000 litre/hr./m²
Capacity of the plant (max.) (12 hrs. working/day)	12000 litres/day
Cost of the plant	Rs. 20000/-
Per capita supply for drinking and cooking	10 litres/day
No. of max. beneficiaries	1200
Operation and maintenance cost	Rs. 4800/- per year
Production cost of water	Rs. 1.11/- per 1000 litre
Contribution per family (calculated on the basis of 240 nos.)	Rs. 2.00/- per month
Arsenic content in raw water	0.19 mg/L
Arsenic content in treated water	BDL to 0.005 mg/L

'Save the Environment' (a Non-Government and non-profit making organisation) has proposed to set up 30 hand-pump attached ARP in six districts of West Bengal in collaboration with Local Govt. Bodies and AIIH&PH, Kolkata.

Removal of Arsenic by the method of activated carbon adsorption technique was also tried in the AIIH&PH laboratory. The laboratory set up was used for filtration through activated carbon bed. Study indicated that though activated carbon could be used for removal of arsenic but economically it would not be feasible.

Removal of arsenic by the method of activated carbon adsorption technique was also tried in the laboratory. The results are presented in Table VI.8.

Ground water with arsenic content was allowed to be filtered at the rate of 1.2 m/h. The performance of activated carbon filter as recorded is presented below 100 gms. of activated carbon was used in the experiment.

Table VI.8: Arsenic Removal by Adsorption Technique

Initial Arsenic Content of Raw Water (mg/L)	Rate of Filtration (m/h)	Recording Time	Arsenic Content in Treated Water
0.08	1	10 a.m.	Nil
0.08	1	11 a.m.	Nil
0.08	1	12 Noon	0.01
0.08	1	1 p.m.	0.02
0.08	1	2 p.m.	0.03
0.08	1	3 p.m.	0.03
0.08	1	4 p.m.	0.05
0.08	1	5 p.m.	0.06
0.08	1	6 p.m.	0.06
0.08	1	7 p.m.	0.07
0.08	1	8 p.m.	0.07

During 10 a.m. to 8 p.m., 6 litres of water was filtered and 0.48 mg of arsenic could be separated out from water through adsorption. The above experiment, however, clearly indicate that though activated carbon could be used for removal of arsenic but economically it would not be feasible. A higher thickness of activated carbon column is necessary to treat higher concentration of arsenic. Charcoal beds were also found to have arsenic adsorption capacity, but with diminished efficiency.

4.3 Method of Exchange

In collaboration with Science and Technology Department, Govt. of West Bengal AIIH&PH carried out study on the efficacy of iodide resin for removal of Arsenic as well as bacterial contamination from water. The study revealed that the iodide resin was effective in removing Arsenic, iron and also bacterial contamination from water.

A filter of diameter 10 cm and length of 40 cm was fabricated with galvanised sheet fitted with controlled inlet and outlet system. Arsenic contaminated water from Ashokenagar was brought to the Sanitary Engineering Deptt. laboratory for carrying out the experimental study. One particular tubewell water was used for the complete study. The three parameters, namely. Arsenic, iron and total and faecal coliform were monitored for evaluating the performance of the polypure system. During the study the water was bacteriologically contaminated by adding domestic sewage as per requirement.

Halogenated resin of 200 gm was-kept over gravel and sand media suitably in the filter to obtain unhindered flow during filtration.

Raw water as well as filtered water quality was monitored during the study. The results are presented in Table VI.9.

Table VI.9: Performance of Halogenated Resin Exchange Media in Domestic Filter for Removal of Arsenic, Iron and Pathogenic Organism from Water

Cumulative Qty. of Raw Water Filtered (lit.)	Rate of Flow (lt/min.)	Arsenic (mg/lit.)		Iron (mg/l)		Total Coliform per 100 ml		Faecal Coliform per 100 ml.	
		Raw	Filtered	Raw	Filtered	Raw	Filtered	Raw	Filtered
10	0.4	0.1269	0.02	3.0	0.04	800	0	300	0
20	0.5	0.1269	0.015	3.0	0.03	2500	0	800	0
30	0.5	0.1269	0.022	3.0	0.04	1800	0	900	0
40	0.1	0.1269	0.021	3.0	0.04	1800	0	900	0
50	0.1	0.1269	0.020	3.0	0.04	1800	0	900	0
60	0.4	0.1269	0.022	3.0	0.04	1000	0	150	0
70	0.1	0.1269	0.021	3.0	0.04	900	0	150	0
80	0.1	0.1269	0.020	3.0	0.04	900	0	150	0
90	0.1	0.1269	0.020	3.0	0.04	900	0	150	0
100	0.1	0.1269	0.020	3.0	0.04	900	0	150	0
125	0.08	0.13	0.010	3.10	0.02	90	0	35	0
150	0.1	0.13	0.025	3.10	0.035	90	0	35	0
175	0.08	0.13	0.020	3.10	0.02	90	0	35	0

Contd...

Table VI.9—Contd...

Cumulative Qty. of Raw Water Filtered (lit.)	Rate of Flow (lt/min.)	Arsenic (mg/lit.)		Iron (mg/l)		Total Coliform per 100 ml		Faecal Coliform per 100 ml.	
		Raw	Filtered	Raw	Filtered	Raw	Filtered	Raw	Filtered
200	0.1	0.13	0.030	3.10	0.04	90	0	35	0
225	0.1	0.13	0.03	3.1	0.05	50	0	17	0
250	0.075	0.125	0.02	2.95	0.05	50	0	17	0
300	0.08	0.125	0.023	2.95	0.06	50	0	17	0
400	0.08	0.125	0.024	2.95	0.07	50	0	17	0
500	0.1	0.11	0.025	2.90	0.10	50	0	17	0
600	0.1	0.11	0.032	2.90	0.10	35	0	11	0
700	0.1	0.11	0.036	2.90	0.11	35	0	11	0
800	0.1	0.11	0.041	2.90	0.11	35	0	11	0
900	0.1	0.13	0.044	2.94	0.12	35	0	11	0
1000	0.1	0.13	0.047	2.94	0.15	30	5	9	0
1100	0.1	0.13	0.049	2.94	0.20	30	7	90	0
1200	0.1	0.13	0.052	2.94	0.30	30	10	90	2

4.3.1 Findings and Discussion

(*a*) Bacteria-removal efficiency of the halogenated resin has been found to be excellent. During the initial period of the study the water was deliberately contaminated with high quantum of total and faecal coliform. The strength and power of halogenated resin to kill bacteria were utilised at a higher rate and as much the presence of total coliform (10/100 ml) and faecal coliform (2/100 ml) in treated water were observed after filtering 1200 litres of highly bacteriologically contaminated water. In this context, it must be mentioned that usually such type of media is used for treatment of water which is bacteriologically contaminated with very low concentration. As such, it can be commented that 200 gm halogenated resin could be used satisfactorily for disinfection of considerable quantum of drinking water.

(*b*) Excellent iron removal in the tune of 98.66 per cent from raw water iron content of 3 mg/L was recorded during initial period of the filtration. The removal efficiency came down to 90 per cent at the final stage of study after filtering 1200 litre of water. The study revealed that 3.24 gm of iron has been effectively removed by the resin media from 1200 litre of water. The present resin media after filtering 1200 litres of water has still capacity to effectively remove iron from considerable quantum of raw water.

(*c*) The halogenated resin media removed arsenic in the tune of 115 mg of Arsenic from 1200 litres of water. The arsenic concentration was brought down below 0.05 mg/L (permissible limit) during the treatment of 1200 litres of water. The effectiveness of halogenated resin deteriorated slightly at faster rate during the filtration due to exchange of iron simultaneously. It can be commented that the same quantum of resin media would show more effectiveness in removal of arsenic if presence of iron remains at lower concentration. As an exchange process the use of halogenated resin is considered to be effective in removal of Arsenic from ground water.

(d) The experimental study was carried out with water having average Arsenic content of 0.13 mg/L. While at the initial stage the arsenic removal efficiency of resin bed was 84.24 per cent, the same at the later stage was found to be decreased to 60 per cent after filtering 1200 litres of contaminated water. The arsenic exchange capacity of the resin bed was found to be reducing slowly with respect to the quantity of water filtered. Iron interfered during the arsenic exchange process in the resin.

(e) By decreasing the rate of filtration from 0.5 lt/min to 0.1 lt/min no appreciable change in Arsenic, iron and coliform organism content in filtrate could be observed at the initial stage. Accordingly the study was carried out maintaining 0.1 lt/min flow rate through the resin media.

(f) As only limited quantity (200 gm) of resin was supplied for the experimental study, the media thickness of 40 mm could be maintained in the experimental set-up. Such thickness of media is considered to be much below the desired media thickness. As such, it is recommended to undertake full scale field demonstration model study with halogenated resin media thickness of 250 mm to 350 mm to explore the economic viability and social acceptability of such unit.

(g) The study was carried out by using only halogenated resin. Polishing resin was not supplied during the study. Accordingly, there was no other alternative but to use single media system for the experimental study. It must be mentioned that multiple resin media bed placed in series would show better performance for removal of arsenic, iron and coliform organism.

(h) It is now recommended to develop hand-pump attached type model unit packed with resin for removal of Arsenic so that it can work at 15 litres/min flow rate. However, such type of units need to be tested further in the field. Home treatment (Filter) unit packed with halogenated resin could be manufactured to explore social acceptability of the unit. As cost is considered to be an important factor, the economic viability of such type of water treatment unit need to be looked into carefully.

Technologies for Arsenic Removal from Drinking Water in Small Communities at Isolated Rural Areas (Year 1997)

Amal K. Datta, Anirban Gupta, Ranjan K. Biswas, Swapan K. Roy and Morshed Alam

Environmental Engineering Laboratory,
Civil Engineering Department, Bengal Engineering College
(Deemed University), Howrah – 711 103

Abstract

A variety of treatment technologies like coagulation, softening, adsorption, and membrane processes have been demonstrated to be effective in removing arsenic from contaminated natural groundwater. However, question remains regarding the efficiency and applicability/appropriateness of the technologies–particularly because of low influent arsenic concentration, and as all the processes are influenced by the source water composition. The present work focuses on the application of one of the above technologies for arsenic removal from drinking water in isolated rural areas.

Introduction

The experts believe that the solution to the arsenic problem in this part of the world lies in the arrangements where:

☆ Use of ground water would be minimized, as far as possible.

☆ The treated surface water would be supplied to the communities in the affected region

☆ Treatment of contaminated ground water for arsenic removal, as short term relief, if no other alternatives are available.

The alternatives are now limited:

1. To leave the contaminated ground water, and to arrange for the supply of surface water after proper treatment,

2. To arrange for the treatment of available contaminated ground water.

However, planning and implementation of schemes for the supply of surface water after proper treatment, require not only a large fund allocation, but also it would take a long period of time. Moreover, nature of soil and want of adequate land area make the process of Rain-Water Harvesting inappropriate in the arsenic affected districts. Therefore measures, like treatment of drinking water for arsenic removal, are recommended as short term relief— which might minimise the agony of the arsenic victims.

People of the arsenic affected areas of this region, where the raw water is derived from either deep wells, or shallow tube wells using hand pumps, are now badly in need of the appropriate technology for the mitigation of the problem. The appropriate technology would definitely be different in three different application areas as follows:

1. Large communities, with existing conventional water treatment plant and piped water supply scheme,

2. Small communities, without any piped water supply system, and

3. Individual Houses in remote and isolated areas.

Suitable strategies for three different application area are listed in Table VI.10.

Technologies for Isolated and Remote Rural Areas

When no other alternative is available, *i.e.*, only when available source is contaminated ground water, arrangement for the removal of arsenic from the drinking water is desirable. Though chemical precipitation is probably the best technology for large scale applications in conventional water treatment plants, the same has been employed successfully in many low cost and easy to operate domestic devices for arsenic removal, and at least in one Well-Head (Hand Pump attached) Unit in this State and their performances are quite satisfactory. Fixed Bed operation, using adsorption is probably the most prospective technology for arsenic removal, in the application area under consideration.

Adoption of a particular technology largely depend on the–

☆ Cost of Installation of the Units, and

☆ Comprehension of the users in respect of the operation and maintenance of the Units.

Table VI.10: Suitable Technologies for Arsenic Removal in Different Application Areas

Application Area	Source: Contaminated Groundwater
Large communities, with piped water supply scheme	Oxidation and Chemical Coagulation; Oxidation and Pressure Filtration with appropriate pre-treatment – in Conventional Water Treatment Plants
Small communities, without any piped water supply system, where the raw water is derived from shallow tube wells, using Hand Pump	Fixed Bed Operation; Oxidation and Chemical Coagulation – in well-head (hand pump attached) units
Individual Houses in remote and isolated areas, where the raw water is also derived from shallow tube wells, using Hand Pumps	Oxidation and Chemical Coagulation Fixed Bed Operation – in domestic units

Merits and demerits of the two above mentioned technologies are presented in Table VI.11.

Fixed Bed Adsorbers

Because of its ease of handling, sludge-free operation and regeneration capability, the fixed bed operation using adsorption and ion exchange techniques has secured a place as one of the popular methods for arsenic removal. Arsenic can be removed by adsorption onto

☆ Activated carbon,

☆ Metal-treated activated carbon,

☆ Oxides and clay minerals,

☆ Activated alumina,

☆ Bauxite, haematite, and feldspar.

☆ Synthetic anion exchange resins,

☆ Chitosan and chitin.

☆ Bone char,

☆ Iron oxide-coated sand (IOCS),

☆ δ-MnO_2-coated sand, etc.

It may be noted that, all the above media can remove arsenic to different extent, and their costs vary widely. However, many of the above media were not field tested; moreover, the process of coating the sand with iron and manganese oxides are cumbersome- unless the coating is done properly, the possibility of detachment of the coating along with the adsorbed arsenic in course of time can not be ruled out. The criteria for selection of one medium should include:

☆ Cost of the medium

☆ Ease or difficulty in operation

Table VI.11: Merits and Demerits of Two Technologies for the Arsenic Removal

Sl.No.	Parameter No.	Fixed Bed Operation using Activated Alumina	Chemical Precipitation Using Chlorine as Oxidant and Aluminium/Iron Salts as Coagulants
1.	Pre-treatment requirement of raw water	No prior treatment of water is required	The raw water is treated first using an oxidant (bleaching powder, chlorine solution, etc.) and a suitable coagulant (iron or aluminium salts)
2.	Cost of Domestic Units	More, as it requires the medium which might cost about Rs. 300.00 over and above the cost of conventional domestic candle filter units. Total cost of installation is around Rs. 650.00 to Rs. 850.00 depending upon the design	Cost is less, as no other component is required other than the conventional domestic candle filter unit
3.	Cost of Installation of Well-Head (Hand Pump Attached) Units	More, well-head units might cost around Rs. 27,000.00 to Rs. 30,000.00, depending upon the engineering design	Cost is less - same as that for conventional water treatment plants for iron removal or coagulation. Low cost modifications would cost lesser
4.	Operation	Simple, as no routine chemical addition is required. High iron content may necessitate occasional washing of the medium - backwash in well-head units	Daily and continuously at least two chemicals are to be added into the raw water before filtration; thereafter, it is settled and filtered to obtain the effluent of acceptable quality

Contd...

Table VI.11–Contd...

Sl.No.	Parameter No.	Fixed Bed Operation using Activated Alumina	Chemical Precipitation Using Chlorine as Oxidant and Aluminium/Iron Salts as Coagulants
5.	Monitoring requirement	Should be monitored at a suitable interval, as the exhausted "medium" should be regenerated and restored by a suitable chemical treatment	Monitoring is not required once it is established that the unit is working
6.	Sludge production	Sludge generates only during the regeneration operation	Sludge generates–every day, and has to be collected and handled carefully by the users
7.	Regeneration process	Consecutive treatment of the medium with 4 per cent NaOH and 0.5N HCl and intermediate wash with water	Does not arise
8.	Disposal of arsenic containing Sludge	Sludge disposal can be done easily at the site of regeneration at controlled condition	The users should be made aware of the consequence of the indiscriminate disposal of arsenic containing sludge; arrangement should be made for their collection and appropriate disposal
9.	Period of continuous operation	One batch of "medium" can be reused several times, after simple chemical treatment for its regeneration and restoration; the attrition and other losses may permit use of one batch of medium for about eight to ten times	Can be used indefinitely with occasional replacement of clogged filter candles

Contd...

Table VI.11–Contd...

Sl.No.	Parameter No.	Fixed Bed Operation using Activated Alumina	Chemical Precipitation Using Chlorine as Oxidant and Aluminium/Iron Salts as Coagulants
10.	Efficiency	Good	Good
11.	Field application	Suitable for small units where daily attention is difficult	Require continuous attention, and as such suitable for large scale use
12.	Infrastructure requirement	Facilities for Monitoring of the Filter Units, and for Regeneration-Restoration of the exhausted media should be developed, before the implementation of any programme. The process of Regeneration-Restoration of the exhausted media is simple and cheap	Facilities for the frequent collection and disposal of sludge has to be developed
13.	Requirement of Supply of Chemicals/ media	Activated alumina of appropriate quality is manufactured in West Bengal, as well as in few other States, and is available in the local market; the production process should be geared up to satisfy the requirement, if the technology is adopted for mass scale application. The chemicals required for regeneration and restoration are easily available and cheap	All the chemicals required for daily operations are easily available and cheap

Table VI.12: Estimated Cost of Well-Head Arsenic Removal Units (Size: 7'3" high × 12" diameter) with Two Different Materials for the Reactor Vessel (Year 1997)

Sl.No.	Item	Amount, Rs.	
		Stainless Steel, 18 SWG, 304 Grade	Polypropylene, glass laminate PPGL (2 mm) with fibre reinforced plastic FRP (3' mm) coating
1.	Reactor Vessel; complete with SS Splash Plate, and other fittings: without flange joint	11,000.00	7,800.00
2.	Supply of Activated Alumina, 100 L	10.000.00	10.000.00
3.	Supply, fitting and fixing of accessories including Force Head Pump, Hand Chemical Pump, Pipe Work, etc.	4,218.00	4,218.00
4.	Material Carrying and Installation Charges including fabrication of MS Stand for Reactor Vessel, MS Stand for PVC Hand Chemical Pump, Supply of Chemicals and charges for Pre-treatment of Media, Building Materials etc.	4,540.00	4.540.00
	Total	**29.758.00**	**26,558.00**

Note: Incidental/Contingent Expenditures and Expenses on Work Charge Establishment are extra.

☆ Cost of operation

☆ Useful Service Life per cycle between regenerations

☆ Potential of reuse (regeneration-restoration)

☆ Regeneration procedure

☆ Number of useful cycles

☆ Possibilities of desorption of absorbed arsenic etc.

In consideration of the above, fixed bed operation through granular activated alumina (AA) appears to be the most promising method for arsenic removal.

The Bengal Engineering College (Deemed University) researchers preferred activated alumina based medium, for fixed bed operations, because of the following advantages:

☆ The medium can be regenerated-restored after its exhaustion

☆ Useful Service Life per cycle between regenerations is pretty long

☆ The medium is manufactured commercially in West Bengal and is available in the local market

☆ Chemicals (*e.g.*, NaOH and HC1) required for Regeneration-Restoration, though technically hazardous, are well known to the common people

Activated Alumina

AAs are mixtures of amorphous and gamma aluminium oxides, prepared by low temperature (300° to 600°C) dehydration of $Al(OH)_3$. The typical AA used in water treatment are of 0.3 to 0.6 mm size. Theoretically, As(III) can not be removed by AA; however, in the study conducted at B.E. College (D.U.). it was observed that the removal capacity of AA for As (III) can be enhanced substantially by treating AA with alkali (4 per cent NaOH) and acid (0.5N HCl) consecutively.

Facility Design

Domestic Arsenic Removal Units

Domestic arsenic removal units, developed at Bengal Engineering College (Deemed University), consist of two chambers, upper one houses the medium (caustic and acid treated AA) and the treated water is collected in the bottom chamber. It was constructed using the-conventional Domestic Candle Filters, from which the ceramic candles were removed and were replaced by a device to produce a desirable rate of flow [in this case. a stainless steel (No. 304) disc with 1 mm aperture]. The volume of medium was 2.75 liters. For easier handling, particularly during regeneration and restoration, the medium was enclosed within nylon bags, with impervious sides and pervious bottom, which could be taken out and subjected to "regeneration restoration" elsewhere, after replacing another bag with fresh medium in the unit. Depending upon the design, the cost of Domestic unit would be Rs. 650.00 to Rs. 850.00. including the cost of the activated alumina. The regeneration-restoration costs Rs. 20.00 each time. Five such Units are field tested in three affected villages in the district of 24-Parganas (N). The performance of the units are commendable in respect of useful service life (more than 8 months)–both in the first cycle and after regeneration-restoration.

Well-Head (Hand-Pump Attached) Units

Basically a Well-head. (Hand-Pump Attached) Arsenic Removal Unit consists of a Reactor Vessel, made of either Stainless Steel or glass laminated polypropylene (PPGL) with fibre reinforced plastic (FRP) lining, or HDPE with FRP lining, and of 300 mm diameter, and 2.2m height supporting about 1300 mm thick layer of activated alumina over a layer of gravel, 200 mm thick, and was operated in the down flow mode. The Units are connected to the existing Tube Wells yielding arsenic contaminated water. The cost of installation of this type of Unit would be about Rs. 27,000.00 to Rs. 30,000.00, depending upon the engineering design; and the cost of regeneration-restoration of the unit is estimated to be around Rs. 700.00 each time (Table VI.12). This type of Well Head Units may serve small rural communities in isolated areas. Two such Well-Head Units, installed at two of the affected villages in the district of 24-Parganas (N), are performing satisfactorily till date, without exhaustion. It may be noted that, till this date, the unit is performing satisfactorily, even after producing more than 2.2 lakh liters (2310 bed volumes) of water. The above unit is serving more than 200 families for the last two and half months.

Disposal of Spent Alkali and Acid Used for Regeneration/ Restoration

The disposal of spent alkali and spent acid, after regeneration/restoration also need special care; the spent alkali is very rich in arsenic. Disposal of spent chemicals, produced during the regeneration-restoration is not a problem, because of the presence of large amounts of dissolved iron in the spent wash- this encourages precipitation of these substances on pH adjustment only. Bengal Engineering College (Deemed University) researchers were able to concentrate the arsenic of spent alkali by simply mixing and adding certain amount of caustic (NaOH), which produced arsenic rich sludge. The supernatant arsenic concentration was either not detectable or very low, which is well within the prescribed limit (US EPA) for direct disposal on ground. The sludge, when dried, confined arsenic in a very small volume, and "stabilization" of this sludge was accomplished using cement (OPC).

Stabilisation of Arsenic-Containing Sludge

The available literature suggests cement-based stabilisation as one of the techniques for the disposal of arsenic containing sludge. Attempts were made to stabilise the arsenic-laden sludge with cement (OPC) and sand. Cement–Sand (1 : 4) mortar specimens using both 5 per cent and 10 per cent (of cement, on dry mass basis) of sludge were tested (Federal EPTox test) for leaching of arsenic from the pulverised mortars, under acidic environment (pH 5 ± 0.5; IN acetic acid). The arsenic concentration of the "leachate" was not detected.

Concluding Remarks

Activated Alumina based Arsenic Removal Units have the potential to provide immediate relief to the affected households in rural West Bengal and Bangladesh, till alternate Water Supply arrangements are made (which in most cases may take a few years). However, the success of the above technology would depend on the creation of infrastructure at villages, for "monitoring" and "regeneration/restoration" of the exhausted media, prior to the distribution of the Filters to the villagers. In respect of maintenance and monitoring requirement. Well-Head units are preferable to the Domestic Arsenic Removal Units.

The following points should be kept in mind while designing and operating an activated alumina-based treatment units:

☆ The spent alkali and spent acid, produced at the time of installation are hazardous, though not toxic and therefore, the two should be mixed for neutralisation before their disposal. Similar care also should be taken for disposal of spent chemicals after regeneration-restoration.

☆ The unit should be provided with a back washing arrangement, which may be needed in view of the high iron content in raw water, and subsequent iron fouling of the bed.

☆ A two-stage treatment–with iron removal in the first stage, followed by activated alumina treatment for polishing would have increased the useful life of the activated alumina. But incidentally, in the iron removal stage too the arsenic will be removed and as such attention is to given in both the stages for the confinement and ultimate disposal of the removed arsenic. The single stage operation, that removes arsenic as well as iron, confines the arsenic in one place, and thus "confinement and ultimate disposal of the removed arsenic" becomes easier. Activated Alumina removes both arsenic and iron. It may also be noted that, substantial removal of iron improves the aesthetic quality of the effluent significantly.

Acknowledgement

The research in B.E. College (D.U.) with activated alumina is being supported by Water for People, Denver, USA. The work was benefited from the advices of Dr. Arun K. Deb, R.F. Weston Inc., USA; Dr. Shanka K. Banerji, University of Missouri-Columbia. USA; Dr. Malay Chaudhuri, IIT, Kanpur; and Dr. Arup K. Sengupta, University of Lehigh, USA. The authors of this paper are indebted to Dr. S.M. Chatterji, Director, and other colleagues in B.E. College (D.U.) for their constant encouragement and co-operation.

Annexure VII
WHO Contribution

During April 29–May 01, 1997 a Regional Consultation was held by the World Health Organisation, South-East Asia Region Office (SEARO), New Delhi on Arsenic in Drinking Water and Resulting Arsenic Toxicity in India and Bangladesh. The following background documents have been published by WHO, SEARO:

Sl.No.	Title	Author	Reference No.
1.	Arsenic management in drinking water	Saumyendra Nath Mukherjee, C.E. (Eastern Zone), PHED, Govt. of West Bengal, Kolkata	SEA/EH/Meet.3/5.3 14 April 1997
2.	Arsenic in Groundwater in Bangladesh	P.L. Smediey, British Geological Survey	SEA/EH/Meet.3/6.1 14 April 1997

Contd...

Sl.No.	Title	Author	Reference No.
3.	Arsenic Pollution in Groundwater in West Bengal, India	Steering Committee Arsenic Investigation Project. PHED, Govt. of West Bengal, Kolkata	SEA/EH/Meet.3/6.2 14 April 1997
4.	Treatment of chronic arsenic toxicity as observed in West Bengal, India	D.N. Guha Mazumder, Prof. and Head, Deptt. of Gastro-enterology IPGME&R, Kolkata	SEA/EH/Meet.3/6.3 14 April 1997
5.	Non-cancer effects of Chronic arsenicosis with special reference to liver damage	D.N. Guha Mazumder, J. Das Gupta, A. Santra, A. Pal, A. Ghose, S. Sarkar, N. Chattopadhyaya and D. Chakraborti	SEA/EH/Meet.3/6.4 14 April 1997
6.	Arsenic calamity due to Groundwater pollution in West Bengal, India	D.N. Guha Mazumder, Dept. of Gastro-enterology, IPGMER, Kolkata	SEA/EH/Meet.3/6.5 14 April 1997
7.	Chronic neuropathy due to arsenic intoxication from geo-chemical source	D. Basu, J. Dasgupta, A. Mukherjee, D.N. Guha Mazumder, Dept. of Neurology and Gastroenterology, IPGMER, Kolkata	SEA/EH/Meet.3/6.6 14 April 1997
8.	Environmental pollution and chronic arsenicosis in South Kolkata, India	D.N. Guha Mazumder, J. Dasgupta, A.K. Chakraborty, A. Chatterjee, D. Das and D. Chakraborti	SEA/EH/Meet.3/6.7 14 April 1997
9.	Chronic arsenic toxicity from drinking tubewell water in rural West Bengal, India	D.N. Guha Mazumder, A.K. Chakraborty, A. Ghose, J.D. Gupta, D. P. Chakraborty, S.B. Dey. and N. Chattopadhyay	SEA/EH/Meet.3/6.8 14 April 1997

Contd...

Sl.No.	Title	Author	Reference No.
10.	Arsenic contamination of groundwater and its remedial action plan in West Bengal, India	Prof. K.J. Nath and Prof. A. Majumder, AIIH&PH, Kolkata	SEA/EH/Meet. 3/6.9 14 April 1997
11.	Guideline value for arsenic in drinking water	Hend Galal-Gorchev, WHO, Geneva	SEA/EH/Meet. 3/6.10 14 April 1997
12.	Arsenic in Groundwater in six districts of West Bengal, India	T.R. Chowdhury, B.Kr. Mandal, G. Samanta, G.Kr, Basu, P.P. Chowdhury, C.R. Chanda, N.Kr. Karan, D. Lodh, R.Kr. Dhar, D. Das, K.C. Saha and D. Chakraborti	SEA/EH/Meet. 3/6.11 21 April 1997
13.	Arsenic in Groundwater in seven districts of West Bengal, India	B.K. Mandal, T.R. Chowdhury, G. Samanta, G.K. Basu, P.P. Chowdhury, C.R.Chanda, D. Lodh, N.K. Karan, R.K. Dhar, D.K. Tamili, D. Das, K.C. Saha and D. Chakraborti	SEA/EH/Meet. 3/6.12 21 April 1997
14.	Arsenic contamination in Groundwater in six districts of West Bengal, India	D. Das, A. Chatterjee, G. Samanta, B. Mandal, T.R. Chowdhury, P.R. Chowdhury, C. Chanda, G. Basu, D. Lodh, S. Nandi, T. Chakraborty, S. Mandal, S.M. Bhattacharya and D. Chakraborti	SEA/EH/Meet. 3/6.13 21 April 1997

Contd...

Sl.No.	Title	Author	Reference No.
15.	Arsenic in Groundwater in six districts of West Bengal, India	A. Chatterjee, D. Das, B.K. Mandal, T.R. Chowdhury, G. Samanta and D. Chakraborti	SEA/EH/Meet. 3/6.14 21 April 1997
16.	Arsenic in Groundwater in six districts of West Bengal, India	D. Das, G. Samanta, B.K. Mandal, T.R. Chowdhury, C.R. Chanda, P.P. Chowdhury, G.K. Basu and D. Chakraborti	SEA/EH/Meet. 3/6.15 21 April 1997
17.	Arsenic in Groundwater– geological review	S.K. Acharyya, DG, GSI	SEA/EH/Meet. 3/5.2 22 April 1997
18.	Arsenic in Groundwater in West Bengal	S.P. Sinha, Ray Director (ER), CGWB, Calcutta	SEA/EH/Meet. 3/6.16 23 April 1997
19.	Excerpts from "Arsenic Contamination of Drinking Water in Bangladesh"	Prof. J.M. Dave	SEA/EH/Meet. 3/6.17 23 April 1997
20.	Excerpts from "Technical Report and Action Plan for Arsenic in drinking water in Bangladesh focussing on health"	Allan H. Smith	SEA/EH/Meet. 3/6.18 23 April 1997
21.	Health effects of arsenic toxicity	Prof. Abdul Wadud Khan, NIPSOM, Dhaka	SEA/EH/Meet. 3/5.1 24 April 1997
22.	Experiences with large scale toxicity in other parts of the world	Allan H. Smith	SEA/EH/Meet. 3/5.5 28 April 1997

Annexure VIII
The Worldwide Arsenic Problems

Drinking water contamination by arsenic and its consequences are described in short according to reports available from different affected countries including-Bangladesh.

Argentina

☆ The first notification of water borne arsenicosis was reported as early as the beginning of this century.

☆ The term "Bell Ville disease" was used to describe arsenic caused skin manifestations among the population of Bell Ville Town.

☆ Several regions in eastern and central Argentina are affected by arsenic in ground water.

☆ Levels often above 100 µg arsenic/L are often found. Even levels above 2000 µg/L have been reported.

☆ The source of contamination was found to be natural due to the soil composition polluting the shallow well waters.

☆ The deeper well water and the surface water showed no or low level of arsenic.

West Bengal, India

☆ The arsenic pollution is of geological origin confined within meander belt zone of the upper delta plain comprising the late quaternary sediment.

☆ Arsenic occurs, at least in part, as arsenopyrite (FeAsS), small proportion of arsenic occur as organic complexes.

☆ The arsenic is mainly found in the groundwater pumped from intermediate depth. As a common rule, aquifers of intermediate depth show above permissible limit of arsenic contents.

☆ High arsenic groundwater is characterised by high iron, calcium, magnesium and bicarbonate. Furthermore by low chloride, sulphate and fluoride.

☆ Seven districts of West Bengal with an area of 37,493000 km^2 inhabited by 34 million people have been surveyed and found to be "at arsenic risk".

☆ 560 villages of 50 blocks out of 162 blocks in the 7 districts are found to be affected with arsenic contamination.

☆ The affected blocks inhabited by 9.6 millions people.

☆ More than 1 million people are drinking water of more than 50 μg arsenic/L.

☆ The average concentration of arsenic in contaminated water is 0.20 mg/L maximum concentration of arsenic is found to be 3.7 mg/L.

☆ 45 per cent of the tested tube wells have arsenic content above 0.05 mg/L.

☆ About 200000 people are showing skin lesions.

☆ Arsenical skin manifestation (melanosis) has been found among the child at the age of 4 years.

☆ In arsenic affected villages, about 20 per cent of the people are showing arsenic lesions.

☆ Another estimate from WHO shows that the number of people drinking, containing more than 50 μg arsenic/L-is as high as 10 million.

Other States, India

Besides West Bengal, cases of arsenic contamination in groundwater have been reported from the States of U.P., Bihar, Jharkhand, North-east hilly states, Chhattisgarh and Punjab. Sporodic cases are reported from Andhra Pradesh, Kerala and Karnataka also.

☆ The number of districts and teh affected population in West Bengal is increasnig with passage of time.

Inner Mongolia, P.R. China

☆ The first case of arsenic poisoning was discovered in 1990.

☆ In 1996, 15 villages of 3 countries were surveyed with respect to pollution health damage.

☆ Many of the arsenic affected areas are located in the arid region (rainfall 2 mm p.a.)

☆ 90 per cent of the wells tested had arsenic at level higher than 50 µg/L.

☆ The highest concentration detected in the well water was 1088 µg/L.

☆ The arsenic contamination is combined with too high concentrations of fluoride.

☆ 35 per cent of 612 checked inhabitants had arsenic lesions.

☆ More serious effects were detected including high cancer mortality.

☆ It was estimated that 655 villages of 11 countries are arsenic affected.

Taiwan

☆ The arsenic problem in Taiwan was reported since 1968, now best known and most studied.

☆ It is Taiwan that gave arsenicosis the name "Black Foot Disease".

☆ Survey of over 83000 wells showed that 19 per cent of the wells had arsenic level 50 µg/L.

☆ 100000 inhabitants drunk water from wells containing 10–1820 µg/L average about 500 µg/L for over 40 years.

☆ On this background a clear dose-response relationships were established on bladder and lung cancer and on bladder cancer mortality.

Thailand

☆ In 1996 arsenic was reported to occur in some shallow as well as deep wells in southern Thailand.

☆ The concentrations found are between 1 and 5100 µg/L. Mexico

☆ 11 countries in the Lagunera Region of northern Mexico have been reported to contain the arsenic problems.

☆ A population of 127000 inhabitants have been drinking water containing 100–500 µg/L.

☆ Various pathological effects, including genotoxic effects of arsenic have been reported.

Chile

☆ Arsenic is not reported to be a problem in 12 of the 13 provinces of Chile.

☆ The arsenic exposure is thus contained in one province, Region II, extending over an area of 125000 km^2 and inhabited by 400000 people.

☆ Antofagusta, the largest city of the region is inhabited by 2/3rd of the region population.

☆ Its water supply utilises three rivers. The water originates from the Andes, brought on aqueducts from upstream sites.

☆ In 1957 and for 12 years to come the drinking water contained 800–1300 µg arsenic/L.

☆ In 1962 the cases of arsenicosis were reported first.

☆ All sorts of specific as well as non specific arsenic intoxications have been reported since 1962.

☆ In 1970 a treatment plant was completed reducing the arsenic contents to 40 µg/L

USA

☆ USA is probably the only (mildly) arsenic affected country which has carried out a nation wide survey of arsenic occurrence in drinking water.

☆ About 347000 people had received public supplied water containing more than 50 µg/L.

☆ About 2.5 million people had received public supplied water containing more than 25 µg/L.

☆ Main arsenic concentration of 46 µg/l was found in one country in California and of 92 µg/L in two countries in Nevada.

☆ Studies from 1972 to 1982 showed to correlation with specific skin alterations and neurological abnormalities.

☆ A case study of recent date has shown increased risk of bladder cancer at very low levels of arsenic exposure in some group.

Bangladesh

☆ The arsenic problems in Bangladesh have only been discovered very recently, the first samples of arsenic contaminated water were analysed as late as in 1993.

☆ Since 1993 the occurrence of arsenic in the ground water has been reported, first and foremost from western bordering districts around the Ganges deltaic plane.

☆ Department of Occupational and Environmental Health (DOEH), NIPSOM first identified arsenicosis cases in Baroghoria Union of Nawabganj district in 1994.

☆ Recently it is discovered that the arsenic contamination also occurs in ground water from outside the Ganges deltaic plain.

☆ 44 districts out of 64 districts of Bangladesh have been found affected with arsenic contamination in ground water. The districts are: Nawabganj, Rajshahi, Natore, Pabna, Meherpur, Kustia, Chuadanga. Jhenaidah, Magura, Rajbari, Faridpur, Narail, Jessore, Satkhira, Madaripur, Shariatpur, Gopalganj, Khulna, Bagerhat, Pirojpur, Barishal, Jhalakathi, Patuakhali, Barguna, Bhola, Manikganj, Narayanganj, Dhaka, Munshiganj, Comilla, Chandpur, Bhahmanbaria, Laxmipur, Noakhali, Feni, Netrokona, Kishoreganj, Narshingdi, Gazipur, Sunamganj, Habiganj, Sythet, Moulavibazar and Kurigram.

☆ The prevalence of arsenicosis have been detected by DOEH, NIPSOM so far concerning 1593 cases in 133 villages of 57 thanas of 26 districts. The districts are: Nawabganj, Rajshahi, Meherpur, Kustia, Khulna, Bagerhat, Jessore, Satkhira, Chuadanga, Jhenaidah, Pabna, Magura, Rajbari, Gopalganj, Faridpur, Laxmipur, Noakhali, Narayanganj, Dhaka, Munshiganj, Narshingdi, Comilla, Chandpur, Gazipur, Kishoreganj, Barishal.

☆ About 3050 tube wells water were analysed by DOEH, NIPSOM. Out of these tube wells 30 per cent have arsenic content above 0.05 mg/L, and 23 per cent have arsenic content in the range of 0.01 to 0.05 mg/L.

☆ The arsenic contamination has been found in shallow tube wells.

☆ Occurrence of arsenicosis is common in the age group of 20–40 years.

☆ The arsenical skin manifestation has also been found at the age of 5 years.

☆ It has been estimated that about 35 millions people are at risk of arsenic toxicity.

Other Countries

In recent years, cases of arsenic pollution in the groundwater have been reported from other countries also such as Vietnam, Nepal and Pakistan.

References

1. MacKenzie, F.T., Lantzy, R.J. and Paterson. V., Global trace metal cycles and predictions. *Journal Int. Assoc. Math. Geol.*, 6: 99–142, 1979.

2. Viraraghavan, T., Jin, Y.C. and. Tonita, P.M., Arsenic in water supplies. *International Journal of Environmental Studies*, 41: 159–167, 1992.

3. Patterson, J.W., *Arsenic in Industrial Wastewater Treatment Technology*, 11–21 Massachusetts: Butterworth Publishers, 1985.

4. Nas, Medical and biologic effects of environmental pollutants: Arsenic, Washington, DC, National Academy of Sciences, 1977.

5. Boyle, R.W. and Jonasson, I.R., The geochemistry of arsenic and its use as an indicator element in geochemical prospecting. *J. Geochem. Explor.*, 2: 251, 1973.

6. Gulbrandsen, R.A., Chemical composition of phosphorites of the phosphoria formation. *Geochim. Cosmochim. Acta*, 30: 769, 1966.

7. Onishi, Y., Arsenic, in *Handbook of Geochemistry*, Vol. 11/3, Wedephol, K.H. Ed., Springer-Verlag, New York, 33–A–1, 1978.

8. Tourtelot, H.A., Minor-element composition and organic carbon content of marine and nonmarine shales of late Cretaceous Age in the western interior of the United States. *Geochim. Cosmochim. Acta*, 28, 1579, 1964.

9. Davis, W.E. *et al.*, In: *Medical and Biologic Effects of Environmental Pollutants: Arsenic*. Washington, DC, National Academy of Sciences, 1971.

10. Cmarko. V., Hygienic problems of arsenic exhalations of ENO plant., *Cesk. Hyg.*, 8: 359–362 (In Slovak, with English summary), 1963.

11. Walsh, L.M. and Keeney, D. R., Behavior and phytotoxicity of inorganic arsenicals in soils. In: Woolson, E. A., ed. *Arsenical Pesticides* Washington, DC, American Chemical Society. (ACS Symp. Ser. No. 7). 1975.

12. Borgona, J.M. and Greiber, R., Epidemiological study of arsenicism in the city of Antofagasta. In: Hemphill, D.D., ed. *Trace Substances in Environmental Health–V*. A Symposium, Columbia, University of Missouri Press, pp. 13–24, 1972.

13. Gonzalez, S.G., In: Memorias del I Simposium International de Laboratorios Veterinarios de Diagnosticos, Mexico, Volume III, pp. 551–560 (in Spanish), 1977.

14. Minkkinen, P. and Yliruokanen, I., The arsenic distribution in Finnish peat bogs, Kemia-kemi, 7–8: 331–335, 1978.

15. Crecelius, E.A., The geochemistry of arsenic and antimony in Puget Sound and Lake Washington, Washington, Thesis, Seattle, Washington, University of Washington, 1974.

16. Johnson, D.L. and Braman, R.S., Alkyl and inorganic arsenic in air samples. *Chemosphere*, 6: 333–338, 1975.

17. Attrep, M., JR. and Anirudhan, M., Atmospheric inorganic and organic arsenic. *Trace Subst. Environ. Health*, 11: 365–369, 1977.

18. Beavington, F. and Cawse, P.A., Comparative studies of trace elements in air particulate in northern Nigeria. *Sci. Total Environ.*, 10: 239–244, 1978.

19. Brimblecombe, P. Atmospheric arsenic. *Nature (Lond.)*, 280: 104–105, 1979.

20. Peirson, D.H., Cawse, P.A. and Cambray, R.S., Chemical uniformity of airborne particulate material and a maritime effect. *Nature (Lond.)*, 251: 675–679, 1974.

21. Walsh, P.R., Duce, R.A. and Fasching, J.L., Impregnated filter sampling system for collection of volatile arsenic in the atmosphere. *Environ. Sci. Technol.*, 11, 163–166, 1977.

22. Braman, R.S. and Foreback, C.C., Methylated forms of arsenic in the environmental. *Science*, 182: 1247–1249, 1973.

23. Ferguson, J.F. and Gavis, J., A review of the arsenic cycle in natural waters. *Water Res.*, 6: 1259–1274, 1972.

24. Durum, W.H., Hem, J.D. and Heidel, S.G., Reconnaissance of selected minor elements in surface waters of the United States, October 1970, Washington, DC, US Department of Interior (Geological Survey Circular 643), 1971.

25. Quentin, K.E. and Winkler, H.A., Occurrence and determination of inorganic polluting agents. *Zentralbl. Bakteriol. (Orig. B)*, 158: 514–523, 1974.

26. Lenvik, K., Steinnes, E. and Pappas, A.C., Contents of some heavy metals in Norwegian rivers. *Nord. Hydrol.*, 9: 197–206, 1978.

27. Borgono, J.M., Vicent, P., Venturino, H. and Infante, A., Arsenic in the drinking water of the city of Antofagasta: epidemiological and clinical study before and after the installation of the treatment plant. *Environ. Health Perspect.*, 19: 103–105, 1977.

28. Clement, W.H. and Faust, S.D., A new convenient method for determining arsenic (+3) in natural waters. *Environ. Lett.*, 5: 155–164, 1973.

29. Penrose, W.R., Conacher, H.B.S., Black, R., Meranger, J.C., Miles, W., Cunningham, H.M. and Squires, W.R., Implications of inorganic/organic interconversion on fluxes of arsenic in marine food webs. *Environ. Health Perspect.*, 19: 53–59, 1977.

30. Onishi, H., Arsenic. In: Wedepohl, K.H., ed. *Handbook of Geochemistry*. Volume, II–2, Chapter 33, Berlin, Springer-Verlag, 1969.

31. Johnson, D.L. and Braman, R.S., The speciation of arsenic and the content of germanium and mercury in members of the Pelagic Sargassum community. *Deep-sea Res.*, 22: 503. 1975.

32. Andreae, M.O., Distribution and speciation of arsenic in natural waters and some marine algae. *Deep-sea Res.*, 25: 391–402, 1978.

33. Johnson, D.L., Bacterial reduction of arsenate in sea water. *Nature (Lond.)*, 240: 44–45. 1972.

34. Harrington, J.M., Middaugh, J.P., Morse, D.L. and Housworth, J., A survey of a population exposed to high concentrations of arsenic in well water in Fairbanks, Alaska. *Am. J. Epidemiol.*, 108: 377–385, 1978.

35. Ritchie, J.A., Arsenic and antimony in some New Zealand thermal waters. *N.Z. J. Sci.*, 4; 218–229, 1961.

36. Nakahara, H., Yanokura, M. and Murakami, Y., Environmental effects of geothermal waste water on the near-by river system. *J. Radioanal. Chem.*, 45: 25–36, 1978.

37. Aggett, J. and Aspell, A.C., Release of arsenic from geothermal sources (New Zealand Energy Research and Development Committee Report No. 35), 1978.

38. Chatterjee, A., Das, D., Mandal, B.K., Choudhury, T.R., Samanta, G. and Chakraborti, D., Arsenic in groundwater in six districts of West Bengal, India: The biggest arsenic calamity in the world. Part 1. Arsenic species in drinking water and urine of the affected people. *Analyst*, 120(3): 643–650, 1995.

39. Das, D., Chatterjee, A., Mandal, B.K., Samanta, G., Chakraborti, D., and Chanda, B., Arsenic in groundwater in six districts of West Bengal, India: the biggest arsenic calamity in the world. Part 2–Arsenic concentration in drinking water, hair, nails, urine,

skin-scale and liver tissue (biopsy) of the affected people. Analyst 120(3): 917–924, 1995.

40. Ramesh, R., Shiv Kumar, K., Eswaramoorthi, S. and Purvaja, G.R., Migration and contamination of major and trace elements in groundwater of Madras City, India. *Environmental Geology*, 25, 126–136. 1995.

41. Grantham, D.G. and Jones, J.F., Arsenic contamination of water wells in Nova Scotia. *Journal American Water Works Association* 69. 653, 1977.

42. Meranger, J.C. and Subramanian, K.S., Arsenic in Nova Scotian groundwater. *The Science of the Total Environment*, 39: 49–55, 1984.

43. Walsh, L.M., Sumner, M.E. and Keeney, D.R., Occurrence and distribution of arsenic in soils and plants. *Environ. Health Perspect.*, 19: 67–71, 1977.

44. Grant, C. and Dobbs, A.J., The growth and metal content of plants grown in soil contaminated by a copper/chrome/arsenic wood preservative. *Environ. Pollut.*, 14: 213–226, 1977.

45. Wauchope, R.D. and McWhorter, C.G., Arsenic residues in soybean seed from simulated MSMA spray drift. *Bull. Environ. Contain. Toxicol.*, 17: 165–167, 1977.

46. Porter, E.K. and Peterson, P.J., Arsenic accumulation by plants on mine waste (United Kingdom). *Sci. Total Environ.*, 4: 365–371, 1975.

47 Andersson, A. and Nilsson, K.O., Enrichment of trace elements from sewage sludge fertilizer in soils and plants. *Ambio*, 1: 176–179, 1972.

48. Furr, A.K., Kelly, W.C., Bache, C.A., Gutenmann, W.H. and Lisk, D.J., Multielement absorption by crops

grown in pots on municipal sludge-amended soil. *J. Agric. Food Chem.,* 24: 889–892, 1976.

49. Lunde, G., Analysis of trace elements in seaweed. *J. Sci. Food Agric.,* 21: 416–418, 1970.

50. Lunde, G., The synthesis of fat and water soluble arseno organic compounds in marine and limnetic algae. *Acta Chem. Scand.,* 27: 1586–1594. 1973.

51. Reay, P.F., The accumulation of arsenic from arsenic-rich natural waters by aquatic plants. *J. Appl. Ecol.,* 9: 557–565, 1972.

52. Pershagen, G., The epidemiology of human arsenic exposure. *Biological and Environmental Effects of Arsenic,* Fowler, B.A. (ed.), 199–232. Amsterdam: Elsevier Science Publishers, 1983.

53. Subramanian, K.S., Arsenic. In: *Quantitative Trace Analysis of Biological Materials,* McKenzie, H.A. and Smythe, L.E. (eds.), 573–587. Amsterdam: Elsevier Science Publishers, 1988.

54. Pontius, F.W., Brown, K.G. and Chen, C.J., Health implications of arsenic in drinking water. *Journal American Water Works Association,* 86, 52–63, 1994.

55. Smith, A.H., Hopenhayn-Rich, C., Bates, M.N., Goeden, H.M., Picciotto, I.H., Duggan, H.M., Wood, R., Kosnett, M.J. and Smith, M.T., Cancer risks from arsenic in drinking water. *Environmental Health Perspectives,* 97: 259–267, 1992.

56. Shen, Y.S., Study of arsenic removal from drinking water. *Journal American Water Works Association,* 65, 543–548, 1973.

57. Chatterjee, A., Das, D. and Chakraborti, D., A study of groundwater contamination by arsenic in the residential area of Behala, Calcutta due to industrial pollution. *Environmental Pollution*, 80: 57–65, 1993.

58. Lianfang, W. and Jianzhong, H., Chronic arsenism from drinking water in some areas of Xinjang, China. In: *Arsenic in the Environment: Part II: Human Health and Ecosystem Effects*, Nriagu, J.O. (ed.). 159–172. New York. N.Y.: John Wiley and Sons, Inc., 1994.

59. American Water Works Association Committee, An AWWA survey of inorganic contaminants in water supplies. *Journal American Water Works Association 77*, 67–72, 1985.

60. Anke, M. Arsenic. *Trace Elements in Human and Animal Nutrition, Volume 2*. Academic Press, Orlando, Fla., 1986.

61. Nielsen, F.H. Nutritional Requirements for Boron, Silicon, Vanadium, Nickel and Arsenic: Current Knowledge and Speculation. *FASEB Jour.*, 5: 12: 2661 (Sept.), 1991.

62. Uthus, E.O. Evidence for Arsenic Essentiality. *Envir. Geo-Chem. and Health*, 14:55, 1992.

63. National Research Council. Recommended Dietary Allowances. National Academy Press, Washington, D.C. (10th ed.), 1989.

64. Abernathy, C.O. Presentation before the AWWA technical Advisory Group, Washington, D.C. (Oct. 25), 1993.

65. Uthus. E.O. Estimation of Safe and Adequate Daily Intake for Arsenic. Risk Assessment of Essential

Elements. Intl. Life Sciences Inst. Press, Washington, D.C., 1994.

66. Mayer, D.R. *et al.* Essential Trace Elements in Humans. Serum Arsenic Concentrations in Hemodialysis Patients in Comparison to Healthy Controls. Biol. Trace Elem. Res., 37:1:27 (Apr.), 1993.

67. Toft, P., Tobin, R.S., Meek, M.E. and Wood, G.C., Guidelines for Canadian drinking water quality. Coping with the Guidelines in the 1990s. In: *Proceedings of the Fourth National Conference on Drinking Water*, Toronto, Ontario, Canada, Sept. 23–25. Tobin, R.S. and Robertson, W.J. (ed.), 1–9, 1990.

68. American Water Works Association Committee. Research needs for inorganic contaminants. *Journal American Water Works Association*, 85, 106–113, 1993.

69. Reid, J., Arsenic occurrence: USEPA seeks clearer picture. *Journal American Water Works Association*, 86, 44–51, 1994.

70. Sayre, I.M., International standards for drinking water. *Journal American Water Works Association* 80, 53–60, 1988.

71. Ginocchio, J.C., Removal of metallic ions during drinking water treatment. *Sulzer Technical Review* 64, 22–26, 1982.

72. Jekel, M.R., Removal of arsenic in drinking water, treatment. In: *Arsenic in the Environment: Part I Cycling and Characterisation*, Nriagu, J.O. (ed.), 119–132. New York: John Wiley and Sons, 1994.

73. International Agency for Research on Cancer. Overall evaluation on carcinogenicity: an updating of IARC

Monographs volumes 1–42, Lyon, 100–106 (IARC Monographs on evaluation of carcinogenic risks to human. Suppl. 7), 1987.

74. Risk assessment forum. Special report on ingested inorganic arsenic skin cancer. Nutritional essentiality. Washington, DC, US Environmental Protection Agency, (EPA–625/3–87/013). 1988.

75. Joint FAO/WHO Expert Committee on Food Additives. Toxicological evaluation of certain food additives and contaminants. Cambridge University Press, 155–162 (WHO Food additives series No. 24), 1989.

76. Ghosh, M.M. and Yuan, J.R. Adsorption of arsenic and organo arsenicals on hydrous oxides. *Environmental Progress*, 6 150–157, 1987.

77. Gupta, S.K. and Chen, K.Y., Arsenic removal by adsorption. *Journal Water Pollution Control Federation*, 50: 493–506, 1978.

78. Edwards, M., Chemistry of arsenic removal during coagulation and Fe-Mn oxidation. *Journal American Water Works Association*, 86, 64–78, 1994.

79. Fowler, B.A., Arsenic metabolism and toxicity to freshwater and marine species. In: *Biological and Environmental Effects of Arsenic*, Fowler, B.A. (ed.), 155–170. Amsterdam: Elsevier Science Publishers, 1983.

80. Aggett, J. and Kriegman, M.R., The extent of formation of arsenic (III) in sediment interstitial waters and its release to hypolimnetic waters in Lake Ohakuri. *Water Res.*, 22(4), 407, 1988.

81. Kohltoff, I.M., Idometric Studes. VII. Reaction between arsenic trioxide and iodine. *Anal. Chem.*, 60, 393, 1921.

82. Ferguson, J.F. and Gavis, J., A review of the arsenic cycle in natural waters. *Water Res.*, 6, 1259, 1972.

83. Glaubig, R.A. and Goldberg, S., Determination of inorganic arsenic (III) and arsenic (III plus V) using automated hydride-generation atomic-absorption spectrometry. *Soil Sci. Soc. Am. J.*, 52. 536. 1988.

84. Haswell, S.J., O'Neill, P. and Bancroft, K.C.C., Arsenic speciation in soil-pore waters from mineralized and unmineralized areas of south-west England, *Talanta*, 32, 69, 1985.

85. Elkhatib, E.A., Bennett, O.L. and Wright, R.J., Kinetics of arsenite sorption in soils. *Soil Sci. Soc. am. J.*, 48, 758, 1984.

86. Lindsay, D.M. and Sanders, J.G., Arsenic uptake and transfer in a simplified estuarine food chain. *Environ. Toxicol. Chem.*, 9, 391, 1990.

87. Kuwabara, J.S., Chang, C.C.Y. and Pasilis, S.P., Effects of benthic flora on arsenic transport. *J. Environ. Eng.*, 116, 394, 1990.

88. Fischer, A.B., Buchet, J.B. and Lauwerys, R.R., Cellular metabolism of arsenic studied in mammalian cells *in vitro*. *Environ. Geochem. Health*, 11, 87, 1989.

89. Andreae, M.O., Determination of arsenic species in natural waters. *Anal. Chem.*, 49, 820, 1977.

90. Walsh, P.R. and Keeney, D.R., Behaviour and phytotoxicity of inorganic arsenicals in soils. In: *Arsenical Pesticides*, Woolson, E.A., Ed., ACS Symp.

Ser. No. 7, American Chemical Society, Washington, D.C., 1975.

91. Lemmo, N.V., Faust. S.D., Belton. T. and Tucker, R., Assessment of the chemical and biological significance of arsenical compounds in a heavily contaminated watershed. I. The fate and speciation of arsenical compounds in aquatic environments: A literature review. *J. Environ. Sci. Health*, 18, 335, 1983.

92. Welch, A.H., Lico, M.S. and Hughes, J.L., Arsenic in groundwater of the western United States. *Ground Water*, 26(3), 333, 1988.

93 Oscarson, D.W., Huang, P.M. and Liaw, W.K., The oxidation of arsenite by aquatic sediments. *J. Environ. Qual.*, 9, 700. 1980.

94. Wood, J.M., Biological cycles for toxic elements in the environment. *Science*, 183, 1049, 1974.

95. Korte, N.E. and Fernando, Q., A review of Arsenic (III) in groundwater. *Critical Reviews in Environmental Control*, 21(1): 1–39, 1991.

96. Matisoff, G., Khourey, C.J., Hall, J.F., Varnes, A.W. and Strain, W.H., The nature and source of arsenic in northeastern Ohio groundwater. *Ground Water*, 20, 446, 1982.

97. Korte, N.E., Naturally Occurring Arsenic in Groundwater at the Kansas City Plant. Environmental Sciences Division Publication #3501, ORNL/TM–11663 Oak Ridge National Laboratory, Grand Junction, CO, 1990.

98. Livesey, N.T. and Huang, P.M., Adsorption of arsenate by soils and its relation to selected chemical properties and anions. *Soil Sci.*, 131(2): 88, 1981.

99. Fuller, C.C., Davis, J.A. and Claypool-Frey, R.G., Partitioning of arsenic by iron oxides in Whitewood Creek, S.D., presented at Division of Environmental Chemistry, American Chemical Society Meeting, Denver, 1987.

100. Johnson, C.A. and Thornton, I., Hydrological and chemical factors controlling the concentrations of Fe, Cu, Zn and As in a river system contaminated by acid mine drainage. *Water Res.*, 21, 359, 1987.

101. Dudas, M.J., Warren, C.J. and Spiers, G.A., Chemistry of arsenic in acid sulphate soils of northern Alberta, Commun. *Soil Sci. Plant Anal.*, 19(7–12), 887, 1988.

102. Jacobs, L.W., Syers, J.K. and Keeney, D.R., Arsenic sorption by soils. *Soils Sci. Soc. Am. J.*, 34, 750, 1970.

103. Wauchope, R.D. and McDowell, L.L., Adsorption of phosphate, arsenate, methanearsenate, cacodylate by lake and stream sediments: Comparisons with soils. *J. Environ. Qual.*, 13, 499, 1984.

104. Davis, J.A., Fuller, C.C., Rea, B.A. and Claypool-Frey, R.G., Sorption and coprecipitation of arsenate by ferrihydrite. In: *Water-Rock Interaction WRI-6*, Miles. D.L., Ed., A.A. Balkema, Rotterdam, 187, 1989.

105 Kingston, F.J., Posner, A.M. and Quirk, J.P., Anion adsorption by goethite and gibbsite II. Desorption of anions from hydrous oxide surfaces. *J. Soil Sci.*, 25, 16, 1974.

106. Moore, J.N., Ficklin, W.H. and Johns, C., Partitioning of arsenic and metals in reducing sulfidic sediments. *Environ. Sci. Technol.*, 22(4), 432, 1988.

107. Mandal, B.K., Roy Chowdhury, T., Samanta, G., Basu, G.K., Chowdhury. P.P., Chanda, C.R., Lodh, D., Karan, N.K., Dhar, R.K., Tamili, D.K., Das, D., Sana. K.C. and Chakraborty, D., Arsenic in groundwater in seven districts of West Bengal, India: The biggest arsenic calamity in the world. *Current Science*, 70(11): 976–986, 1996.

108. NEERI Technical Digest No. 56, Arsenic determination in drinking water, April, 1977.

109. NEERI Technical Digest No.82. Determination of low levels of arsenic in drinking waters (January), 1988.

110. Pande, S.P. and Hasan, M.Z., Improved method for determination of arsenic in water. *Ind. J. Env. Hlth.,* 20(2): 121, 1978.

111. Pande, S.P. and Hasan, M.Z., New solvent for SDDC in determination of arsenic. *Ind. J. Env. Hlth.,* 21: 332, 1979.

112. Pande, S.P. and Sarin, R., Determination of nanogram levels of arsenic in drinking water. *Ind. J. Env. Hlth.,* 22(1): 187, 1980.

113. Pande, S.P., Morpholine as a new substitute for pyridine in the determination of arsenic in water. *J. Inst. Chemists (India)*, 52: 256, 1980.

114. Pande, S.P., Arsenic in aquatic, environment: A review. *Chemical Bra*, 19(4): 99, 1983.

115. Chakraborti, D., Valentova, M. and Sucha, L. Prague Inst. Chem. Technol. Czechoslovakia Analyst. Chem., H–17: 31–42, 1982.

116. Chatterjee, A., Das, D., Mandal, B.K., Roy Chowdhury, T., Samanta, G. and Chakraborti, D., *Analyst*, 120: 643–650, 1995.

117. Das, D., Chatterjee, A., Mandal, B.K., Samanta, G., Chanda, B. and Chakraborti, D., *Analyst*, 120": 917–924, 1995.

118. Fox, K.R. and Sorg, T.J., Controlling arsenic, fluoride and uranium by point of use treatment. *Journal American Water Works Association*, 79: 81–84, 1987.

119. Rozelle, L.T., Point of use and point of entry drinking water treatment. *Journal American Water Works Association*, 79: 53–59, 1987.

120. United States Environmental Protection Agency (USEPA), *Manual of Treatment Techniques for Meeting the Interim Primary Drinking Water Regulations*, EPA–600/8–77–005. S.I.: USEPA, 1978.

121. Logsdon, G.S. and Symons, J.M., Removal of trace inorganics by drinking water treatment unit processes. *AICHE Symposium Series*, 70: 367–377, 1973.

122. Logsdon, G.S., Sorg, T.J. and Symons, J.M., Removal of heavy metals by conventional treatment. In: *Proceedings 16th Water Quality Conference on Trace Metals in Water Supplies: Occurrence, Significance and Control*, 111–133. Urbana Champaign, Illinois: University of Illinois, Urbana Champaign, 1993.

123. Clifford, D., Subramanian. S. and Sorg, T.J., Removing dissolved inorganic contaminants from water. *Environmental Science and Technology*, 20: 1072–1080, 1993.

124. Chang, S.D., Ruiz, H., Bellamy, W.D., Spangenberg, C.W. and Clark, D.L., Removal of arsenic by enhanced coagulation and membrane technology: Critical Issues in Water and Wastewater Treatment. In: *Proc. of the 1994 National Conference on Environmental Engineering.* Boulder, Colorado, July 11–13, 1994.

125. Krapf, N.E., Commercial scale removal of arsenite, arsenate and methyl arsenate from ground and surface water. In: *Arsenic: Industrial, Biomedical and Environmental Perspectives.* Lederer, W.H. and Fensterheim, R.J. eds. 269–281. New York: Van Nostrand Reinhold, 1963.

126. Lauf, G.F. and Waer, M.A., *Arsenic Removal Using Potassium Permanganate,* Miami, Florida: AWWA–WQTC, 1993.

127. Harper, T.R. and Kingham, N.W., Removal of arsenic from wastewater using chemical precipitation methods. *Water Environment Research,* 64, 200–203, 1992.

128. Brewster, M.D., Removing arsenic from contaminated wastewater. *Water Environment and Technology,* 54–57, 1992.

129. Kanbar, S.A., Arsenic Removal from Drinking Water in the Presence of Iron, *Doctoral Thesis,* New Mexico State University, Las Cruces, New Mexico, 1983.

130. Rajakovic, L.V., Mitrovic, M.V., Stevanovic, S.M. and Dimitrijevic, S.P., Comparative study of arsenic removal from drinking water (precipitation, sorption and membrane processes). *Journal of the Serbian Chemical Society,* 58: 131–143, 1993.

131. Rajakovic, L.V. and Mitrovic, M.M., Arsenic removal from water by chemisorption filters. *Environmental Pollution*, 75: 279–287. 1992.

132. Cooper, K.H. and Thompson, R.E., Iron, manganese and arsenic removal using high-rate adsorption clarification-mixed media filtration process. In: *Proceedings AWWA Annual Conference*, Cincinnati, Ohio, USA, 1147–1166. 1990.

133. Sorg, T.J. and Logsdon, G.S., Treatment technology to meet the interim primary drinking water regulations for inorganics: Part 2. *Journal American Water Works Association*, 70: 379–393, 1978.

134. Gulledge, J.H. and O'connor, J.T., Removal of arsenic (V) from water by adsorption on aluminium and ferric hydroxides. *Journal American Water Works Association*, 65: 548–552, 1973.

135. Cheng, R.C., Liang, S., Wang, H.C. and Beuhler, M.D., Enhanced coagulation for arsenic removal. *Journal American Water Works Association*, 86(9): 79–90, 1994.

136. Maruyama, T., Hannah, S.A. and Cohen, J., Metal removal by physical and chemical treatment processes. *Journal Water Pollution Control Federation*, 47: 962–975, 1975.

137. Dutta, A. and Chaudhuri, M., Removal of arsenic from groundwater by lime softening with powdered coal additive. *Aqua*, 40: 25–29, 1991.

138. Fox. K.R., Field experience with point of use treatment systems for arsenic removal. *Journal American Water Works Association*, 81: 94–101, 1989.

139. Hathaway, S.W. and Rubel, P., Removing arsenic from drinking water. *Journal American Water Works Association*, 79(8): 61–65, 1987.

140. Bellack, E., Arsenic removal from potable water. *Journal American Water Works Association*, 63: 454–458, 1971.

141. Cox, C.D. and Ghosh, M.M., Surface complexation of methylated arsenates by hydrous oxides. *Water Research*, 28: 1181–1188, 1994.

142. Clifford, D., Ion exchange and inorganic adsorption. *Water Quality and Treatment: A Handbook of Community Water Supplies*, 561–633. New York: McGraw-Hill, 1990.

143. Cox, C.D., Ghosh, M.M. and Teoh, R.S., Sorption of organo arsenicals on clay and hydrous oxide surfaces, In: *Proceedings of the 1988 Joint CSCE–ASCE National Conference*, July 13–15, Vancouver, B.C., 401–408, 1988.

144. Sigworth, E.A. and Smith, S.B., Adsorption of inorganic compounds by activated carbon. *Journal American Water Works Association*, 64: 386–391, 1972.

145. Diamadopoulos, E., Samaras, P. and Sakellaropoulos, G.P., The effect of activated carbon properties on the adsorption of toxic substances. *Water Science and Technology*, 25: 153–160, 1992.

146. Elson, C.M., Davies, D.H. and Hayes, E.R., Removal of arsenic from contaminated drinking water by a chitosan/chitin mixture. *Water Research*, 14: 1307–1311, 1980.

147. Hiavay, J., Foldi-Polyak, K. and Pataki. K., Removal of toxic metals from natural water by adsorption method. In: *Proceedings of the 4th Conference on Applied Chemistry, Unit Operations and Processes*, 72–77 Budapest: Hungarian Chemical Society, 1983.

148. Huang, C.P. and Fu, P.L.K., Treatment of arsenic (V)-containing water by the activated carbon process. *Journal Water Pollution Control Federation*, 56. 233–242, 1984.

149. Huang, C.P. and Vane, L.M., Enhancing As(V) removal by a Fe(II)–treated activated carbon. *Journal Water Pollution Control Federation*, 61: 1596–1603, 1989.

150. Guha, S. and Chaudhuri, M., Removal of arsenic III from groundwater by low-cost materials. *Asian Environment*, 12(1), 42–50, 1990.

151. Singh, D.B., Prasad, G., Rupainwar, D.C. and Singh, V.N., As III removal from aqueous solution by adsorption. *Water, Air and Soil Pollution*, 42: 373–386, 1989.

152. Prasad, G., Removal of arsenic V from aqueous systems by adsorption onto some geological materials. In: *Arsenic in the Environment Part I: Cycling and Characterization*, Nria-gu. J.O. (ed.), 133–154. New York: John Wiley and Sons, 1994.

153. Chanda, M., O'Driscoll, K.F. and Rempel, G.L., Ligand exchange sorption of arsenate and arsenite anions by chelating resins in ferric ion form–I. Weak-base chelating resin Dow XFS–4195. *Reactive Polymers*, 7: 261, 1988.

154. Chanda, M., O'Driscoll, K.F. and Rempel, G.L., Ligand exchange sorption of arsenate and arsenite anions by chelating resins in ferric ion form–II. Iminodiacetic chelating resin chelex 100. *Reactive Polymers*, 8: 85–95. 1988.

155. Huxstep, M.R., Inorganic contaminant removal from drinking water by Reverse Osmosis, USEPA Report No. EPA-600/2-81-115. Florida: USEPA, 1981.

156. Magyar, J., Kelliher Arsenic Removal Study: Final Report to Saskatchewan Environment and Public Safety Department, 1992.

157. Phommavong. T. and Viraraghvan, T., Arsenic removal by manganese greensand filters. In: *Proceedings of the 1994 National Conference on Environmental Engineering (American Society of Civil Engineers)*, Ryan, J.N. and Edwards, M. (eds.), Denver, Colorado, 646–653, 1994.

158. Lauf, G.F., Arsenic removal using potassium permanganate generated greensand. In: *Proceedings. AWWA–WQTC Conference*, San Francisco, California, 1994.

159. ADI Limited, Research Study into Arsenic Removal from Groundwater, (Document No. 18). Fredericton, New Brunswick: ADI Limited, 1993.

160. Driehaus, W., Seith, R. and Jekel, M., Oxidation of arsenic (III) with manganese oxides in water treatment. *Water Research*, 29(1): 297–305, 1995.

161. Trace Inorganic Substances Research Committee, American Water Works Association (AWWA), A review of solid-solution interactions and implications

for the control of trace inorganic materials in water treatment. *Journal of American Water Works Association*, 80: 56–64, 1988.

162. Clifford, D., Processes for removal of inorganic contaminants from water. *Water Engineering and Management' Reference Handbook*, 31–38, 1982.

163. Faust, S.D. and Aly, O.M., *Chemistry of Water Treatment*. Massachusetts: Butterworth Publishers, 1983.

164. McDonald, R.A., McLeod, B.R. and Rosenfeld, J.E., Treatment options for Specific contaminants. In: Guidelines for Canadian Drinking Water Quality: Water Treatment Principles and Applications– A Manual for the Production of Drinking Water, 230–231. Canada: National Health and Welfare, 1993.

165. Sorg, T.J. and Logsdon, G.S., Treatment technology to meet the interim primary drinking water regulations for inorganics: Part 5, *Journal of American Water Works Association*, 72: 411, 1980.

166. Willey, B.R., Finding treatment options for inorganics. *Water Engineering and Management*, 134: 28–31, 1987.

167. Hsia, T.H. and Lo, K.L., The pollution problems and treatment methods of arsenic in water. *Water Supply*, 8 (3/4), 32–44. 1994.

168. Hamann, C.L., McEwan, J.B. and Myers, A.G., Guide to selection of water treatment processes, American Water Works Association, Water Quality and Treatment: A Handbook of Community Water Supplies, Fourth Edition, Pontius, F.W. (ed.) 157–186: McGraw-Hill. Inc., 1994.

169. Aggett, J. and Kriengman, M.R., Preservation of arsenic (III) and arsenic (V) in samples of sediment interstitial water. *Analyst*, 112: 153, 1987.

170. Tallman, D.E. and Shaikh, A.U., Redox stability of inorganic arsenic (III) and arsenic (V) in aqueous solution. *Anal. Chem.*, 52: 196, 1980.

171 Seyler, P. and Martin, J.-M., Biogeochemical processes affecting arsenic species distribution in a permanently stratified lake. *Environ. Sci. Technol.*, 23: 1258, 1989.

172. Feldman, C., Improvements in the arsine accumulation-helium glow detector procedure for determining traces of arsenic. *Anal. Chem.*, 51(6): 664, 1979.

173. Aggett, J. and O'Brien, G.A., Detailed model for the mobility of arsenic in lacustrine sediments based on measurements in Lake Ohakuri. *Environ. Sci. Technol.*, 19: 231, 1985.

174. Faust, S.D., Winka, A.J. and Belton, T., An assessment of chemical and biological significance of arsenic species in the Maurice River drainage basin (N.J.). I. Distribution in water, river and lake sediments. *J. Environ. Sci. Health*, 22: 209, 1987.

175. Faust, S.D., Winka, A.J. and Belton, T., An assessment of chemical and biological significance of arsenical species in the Maurice River drainage basin (N.J.). II: Partitioning of arsenic into bottom sediments. *J. Environ Sci. Health*, 22: 239, 1987.

176. Brockbank, C.I., Batley, G.E. and Low, G.K.C., Photochemical decomposition of arsenic species in natural waters. *Environ. Technol. Lett.*, 9: 1361, 1988.

177. Oscarson, D.W., Huang, P.M. and Liaw, W.K., Role of manganese in the oxidation of arsenite by freshwater lake sediments, Clay. *Clay Min.*, 29: 219, 1981.

178. Vogel, A.E., *A Textbook of Macro and Semimacro Qualitative Inorganic Analysis*, 4th edn., London, Longmans, 1955.

179. Vasak, V. and Sedivec, V., The colorimetric determination of arsenic. *Chem. Listy*, 46: 341–344, 1952.

180. Stratton, G. and Whitehead, H.C., Colorimetric determination of arsenic in water with silver diethyldithiocarbamate. *J. Am. Water Works Assoc.*, 54: 861–864, 1962.

181. Gastiner, E., On the spectrophotometric determination of arsenic using silver diethyl-thiocarbamidate. *Mikrochim. Acta*, 526–543 (in German), 1972.

182. Hundley, H.K. and Underwood, J.C., Determination of total arsenic in total diet samples. *J. Assoc. Off. Anal. Chem.*, 53: 1176–1178, 1970.

183. Kopp, J.F., 1-Ephedrine in chloroform as a solvent for silver diethyl-dithiocarbamate in the determination of arsenic. *Anal. Chem.*, 45: 1786–1787, 1973.

184. Sandhu, S.S. and Nelson, P., Ionic interference in the determination of arsenic in water by the silver diethyldithiocarbamate method. *Anal. Chem.*, 50: 322–325, 1978.

185. Portmann, J.E. and Riley, J.P., Determination of arsenic in sea water, marine plants and silicate and carbonate sediments. *Anal. Chim. Acta.* 31: 509–519, 1964.

186. Johnson, D.L. and Pilson, M.E.Q., Spectrophotometric determination of arsenite, arsenate and phosphate in natural waters. *Anal. Chim. Acta*, 48: 289, 1972.

187. Holak, W., Gas-sampling technique for arsenic determination by atomic absorption spectroscopy. *Anal. Chem.*, 41: 1712–1713, 1969.

188. Kirkbright, G.F. and Ranson, L., Use of the nitrous oxide-acetylene flame for determination of arsenic and selenium by atomic absorption spectrometry. *Anal. Chem.*, 43: 1238–1241, 1971.

189. Menis, O. and Rains, T.C., Determination of arsenic by atomic absorption spectrometry with electrodeless discharge lamp as source of radiation. *Anal. Chem.*, 41: 952–954, 1969.

190. Ando, S., Suzuki, M., Fuwa, K. and Vallee, B. L., Atomic absorption of arsenic in nitrogen (entrained air) hydrogen flames. *Anal. Chem.*, 41: 1974–1979, 1969.

191. Siemer, D.D. and Koteel, P., Comparisons of methods of hydride generation atomic absorption spectrometric arsenic and selenium determination. *Anal. Chem.*, 49: 1096–1099, 1977.

192. Smith, D.C., Leduc, R. and Tremblay, L., Pesticide residues in the total diet in Canada. IV. 1972 and 1973. *Pestic Sci.*, 6: 75–82, 1975.

193. Griffin, H.R., Hocking, M.B. and Lowery, D.G., Arsenic determination in tobacco by atomic absorption spectrometry. *Anal. Chem.*, 47: 229, 1975.

194. McDaniel, M., Shendrikar, A.D., Reiszner, K.D. and West, P.W., Concentration and determination of

selenium from environmental samples. *Anal. Chem.*, 48: 2240–2243, 1976.

195. Siemer, D.D., Koteel, P. and Jariwala, V., Optimization of arsine generation in atomic absorption arsenic determinations. *Anal. Chem.*, 48: 836–840, 1976.

196. Heydorn, K. and Damsgaard, E., Simultaneous determination of arsenic, manganese and selenium in biological materials by neutron-activation analysis. *Talanta*, 20: 1–11, 1973.

197. Maruyama, Y. and Komiya, K., Determination of copper, arsenic and mercury in tobacco leaves by neutron activation analysis. *Radio-isotopes*, 5: 279, 1973.

198. Orvini, E., Gills, T.E. and LaFleur, P.D., Method for determination of selenium, arsenic, zinc, cadmium and mercury in environmental matrices by neutron activation analysis. *Anal. Chem.*, 46: 1294–1297, 1974.

199. Takeo, T. and Shibuya, M., Determination of arsenic in tea plant by neutron activation analysis. *Nippon Shokuhin Kogyo Gakkai-Shi*, 19(2): 91, 1972.

200. Raby, B.J. and Johnson, D.L., A method for the neutron activation analysis of natural waters for arsenic. *Anal. Chim. Acta*, 62: 196–199, 1972.

201. Gallorini, M., Greenberg, R.R. and Gills, T.E., Simultaneous determination of arsenic, antimony, cadmium, chromium, copper and selenium in environmental material by radiochemical neutron activation analysis. *Anal. Chem.*, 50: 1479–1481, 1978.

202. Arnold, J.P. and Johnson, R.M., Polarography of arsenic. *Talanta*, 16: 1191–1207, 1969.

203. Davis, P.H., Dulude, G.R., Griffin, R.M., Matson, W.R. and Zink, E.W. Determination of total arsenic at the nanogram level by high-speed anodic stripping voltammetry. *Anal. Chem.*, 50: 137–143, 1978.

204. Myers, D.J. and Osteryoung, J., Determination of arsenic (III) at the parts per billion level by differential pulse polarography. *Anal. Chem.*, 45: 267–271, 1973.

205. Eiton, R.K. and Geiger, W.E., Analytical and mechanistic studies of the electrochemical reduction of biologically active organoarsenic acids. *Anal. Chem.*, 50: 712–717, 1978.

206. Braman, R.S., Johnson, D.L., Foreback, C.C., Ammons, J.M. and Bricker, J.L., Separation and determination of nano-gram amounts of inorganic arsenic and methylarsenic compounds. *Anal. Chem.*, 49: 621–625, 1977.

207. Kirkbright, G.F., Ward, A.F. and West, T.S., Atomic emission spectrometry with an induction–coupled high frequency plasma source. The determination of iodine, mercury, arsenic and selenium. *Anal. Chim. Acta*, 64: 353, 1973.

208. Robbins, W.B., Caruso, J.A. and Fricke, F.L., Determination of germanium, arsenic, selenium, tin and antimony in complex samples by hydride generation-microwave-induced plasma atomic-emission spectrometry. *Analyst*, 104: 35–40, 1979.

209. Thomson, K.C., The atomic-fluorescence determination of antimony, arsenic, selenium and tellurium by using the hydride generation technique. *Analyst*, 100: 307–310, 1975.

210. Zeman, A., Ruzicka, J., Stary, J. and Kleckova, E., A new principle of activation analysis separations. VII. Substoichiometric determination of traces of arsenic. *Talanta*, 11: 1143, 1964.

211. Carvalho, M.B. and Hercules, D.M., Trace arsenic determination by volatilization and X-ray photoelectron spectroscopy. *Anal. Chem.*, 50: 2030–2034, 1978.

212. Goode, S.R. and Mattews, R.J., Enzyme-catalyzed reaction-rate method for determination of arsenic in water. *Anal. Chem.*, 50: 1608–1610, 1978.

213. Lauwerys, R.R., Buchet, J.P. and Roels, H., The determination of trace levels of arsenic in human biological materials. *Arch. Toxicol.*, 41: 239–247, 1979.

214. Crecelius, E.A., Changes in the chemical speciation of arsenic following ingestion by man. *Environ, Health Perspect.*, 19: 147–150, 1977.

215. Andreae, M.O., Determination of arsenic species in natural waters. *Anal. Chem.*, 49: 820–825, 1977.

216. Feldman, C. and Batistoni, D.A., Spectroscopic element detector for gas chromatography. *Anal. Chem.*, 49: 2215–2221, 1977.

217. Crecelius, E.A., Modification of the arsenic speciation technique using hydride generation. *Anal. Chem.*, 50: 826–827, 1978.

218. Talmi, Y. and Norvell, V.E., Determination of arsenic and antimony in environmental samples using gas chromatography with a microwave emission spectrometric system. *Anal. Chem.*, 47: 1510–1516, 1975.

219. Soderquist, C.J., Crosby, D.G. and Bowers, J.B., Determination of cacodylic acid (hydroxy-dimethylarsine oxide) gas chromatography. *Anal. Chem.*, 46: 155–157, 1974.

220. Edmonds, J.S., Francesconi, K.A., Cannon, J.R., Raston, C.L., Skelton, B.W. and White, A.H., Isolation, crystal structure and synthesis of arsenobetaine, the arsenical constituent of the western rock lobster Panulirus Longipes Cygnus George. *Tetrahedron Lett.*, 18: 1543–1546, 1977.

221. Cooney, R.V., Mumma, R.O. and Benson, A.A., Arsoniumphos-pholipid in algae. *Proc. Nat. Acad. Sci.*, 75: 4262–4264, 1978.

222. Lunbde, G., Occurrence and transformation of arsenic in the marine environment. *Environ. Health Perspect.*, 19: 47–52, 1977.

223. Sturgeon, R.E., Siu, K.M.W., Willie, S.N. and Berman, S.S., Quantification of arsenic species in a river water reference material for trace metals by graphite furnace atomic absorption spectrometric techniques. *Analyst*, 114: 1393, 1989.

224. Ridley, W.P., Dizikes, I.J. and Wood. J.M., Biomethylation of toxic elements in the environment. *Science*, 197: 329, 1977.

225. Yamamoto, M., Determination of arsenate, methanearsonate and dimethylarsinate in water and sediment extracts. *Soil Sci. Soc. Am. Proc.*, 39: 859, 1975.

226. Kopp, J.F., "1-Ephedrine in chloroform as a solvent for silver diethyldithiocarbamate in determination of arsenic, *Anal. Chem.*, 45: 1786, 1973.

227. American Public Health Association, *Standard Methods for the Examination of Water and Wastewater*, 13th Ed., American Public Health Association. Washington, D.C., 62, 1971.

228. Clement, W.H. and Faust, S.D., A new convenient method for determining arsenic (+3) in natural waters. *Environ. Lett.*, 5: 155, 1973.

229. Peoples, S.A., Lasko, J. and Lais, T., The simultaneous determination of methylarsonic acid and inorganic arsenic in urine. *Proc. West. Pharmacol. Soc.*, 14: 178, 1971.

230. Fernandez, F.J., Atomic absorption determination of gaseous hydrides utilizing sodium borohydride reduction. *Atomic Absorption Newsl.*, 12: 93, 1973.

231. Schmidt, F.J. and Royer, I.L., Sub-microgram determination of arsenic, selenium, antimony and bismuth by atomic absorption utilizing sodium borohydride reduction. *Anal. Lett.*, 6: 17, 1973.

232. Aggett, J. and Aspell, A.C., The determination of arsenic (III) and total arsenic by atomic absorption spectroscopy, *Analyst*, 101: 341, 1976.

233. Braman, R.S. and Foreback, C.C., Methylated forms of arsenic in the environment. *Science*, 182: 1247. 1973.

234. Knudsen, E.J. and Christian, G.D., Flameless atomic absorption determination of volatile hydrides using cold trap collection. *Anal. Lett.*, 6: 1039, 1973.

235. Lussi-Schlatter, B. and Brandenberger, H., Trace detection of some inorganic hydrides such as arsine. germanium hydride, stibine and tin hydride by gas chromatography with mass specific detection. In:

Advances in Mass Spectrometry in Biochemistry and Medicine, Vol. 2, Spectrum Publications, Laurel, MD, 1976, 231.

236. Van Wagenen, S., Carter, D.E., Ragheb, A.G., and Fernando, Q., Kinetic control of peak shapes in atomic absorption arsenic determinations by arsine generation. *Anal. Chem.,* 59: 891, 1987.

237. Grabinski, A.A., Determination of arsenic (III), arsenic (V), monomethylarsonate and dimethylarsinate by ion-exchange chromatography with flameless atomic absorption spectrometric detection. *Anal. Chem.,* 53: 966, 1981.

238. Hinners, T.A., Arsenic speciation: Limitations with direct hydride analysis. *Analyst,* 105: 751, 1980.

239. Howard, A.G. and Arbab-Zavar, M.H., Determination of "inorganic" arsenic(III) and arsenic(V), "Methylarsenic" and "dimethylarsenic" species by selective hydride evolution atomic absorption spectroscopy. *Analyst,* 106: 213, 1981.

240. Boampong, C., Brindle, I.D. and Ceccarelli-Ponzoni, C.M., Determination of arsenic by hydride generation in the D.C. plasma atomic emission spectrometer: determination of arsenic (III) and arsenic (V) as total arsenic. *J. Anal. Atomic Spectrom.,* 2: 197, 1987.

241. Panaro. K.W. and Krull, I.S., Continuous hydride generation with direct current plasma emission spectroscopic detection for total arsenic determinations. *Anal. Lett.,* 17: 157, 1984.

242. Thompson, M., Pahlavanpour, B., Walton, S.J. and Kirk-bright, G.F., Simultaneous determination of trace

concentrations of arsenic, antimony, bismuth, selenium and tellurium in aqueous solutions by introduction of the gaseous hydrides into an inductively coupled plasma source for emission spectrometry. I. *Analyst*, 103: 705, 1978.

243 Thompson, M., Pahlavanpour, B., Walton, S.J. and Kirkbright, G.F., Simultaneous determination of trace concentrations of arsenic, antimony, bismuth, selenium and tellurium in aqueous solutions by introduction of the gaseous hydrides into an inductively coupled plasma source for emission spectrometry. II. *Analyst*, 103(1227): 568, 1978.

244. Liddle, J.R., Brooks, R.R. and Reeves, R.D., Some parameters affecting hydride generation from arsenic(V) for atomic absorption spectrophotometry. *J. Assoc. Off. Anal. Chem.*, 63: 1175, 1980.

245. Arbab-Zavar, M.H. and Howard, A.G., Automated procedure for the determination of soluble arsenic using hydride generation atomic-absorption spectroscopy. *Analyst*, 150: 744, 1980.

246. Hershey, J.W. and Keliher, P.N., Some hydride generation inter-element interference studies utilizing atomic absorption and indictively coupled plasma emission spectrometry. *Spectrochim. Acta*, 41B: 713, 1986.

247. Welz, B. and Melcher, M., Mechanisms of transition metal interferences in hydride generation atomic absorption spectrometry. II. *Analyst*, 109, 573, 1984.

248. Welz, B. and Melcher, M., Mechanisms of transition metal interferences in hydride generation atomic absorption spectrometry. III. *Analyst*, 109: 577, 1984.

249. Welz, B. and Schubert–Jacobs, M.J., Mechanisms of transition metal interferences in hydride generation atomic absorption spectrometry. IV, J. Anal. Spectrosc., 1, 23, 1987.

250. Aggett, J. and Hayashi, Y., Observations on the interference by copper (II), cobalt (II) and nickel (II) on the determination of arsenic by arsine generation atomic absorption spectrometry. Analyst, 112, 277, 1987.

251. Dornemann, A. and Kleist, H., Hydridmethode zur Arsenbestim–mung durch Atomabsorptions Speaktrometric mit Atomisicrung in Heissen Quartzrohs, Fresenius' Z. Anal. Chem., 305. 379, 1981.

252. Boampong, C., Brindle, I.D., Le, X.C., Pidwerbesky, L. and Ceccarelli-Ponzoni, C.M., Interference reduction by L-cystine in the determination of arsenic by hydride generation. *Anal. Chem.*, 60: 1185, 1988.

253. Ediger, R., Atomic absorption analysis with the graphite furnace using matrix modification. *Atomic Absorption Newsl.*, 14: 127, 1975.

254. Walsh, P.R., Fasching, J.L. and Duce, R.A., Losses of arsenic during the low temperature ashing of atmospheric particulate samples. *Anal. Chem.*, 48: 1012, 1976.

255 Iverson, D.G., Anderson, M.A., Holm, T.R., Stanforth, R.R., An evaluation of column chromatography and flameless absorption spectrophotometry for arsenic speciation as applied to aquatic systems. *Environ. Sci. Technol.*, 13: 1491, 1979.

256. Henry, F.T. and Thorpe, T.M., Determination of arsenic (III) and arsenic (V) by differential pulse polarography after separation by ion exchange. *Anal. Chem.*, 52: 80, 1980.

257. Dietz, E.A., Jr., Perez, M.A., Purification and analysis methods for methylarsonic acid and hydroxy-dimethylarsine oxide. *Anal. Chem.*, 48: 1088, 1976.

258. Dhankher, P., Li,Y., Rosen, B.P., Shi, J., Salt, D., Senecoff, J.F., Sashti, N.A. and Meagher, R.B., Engineering tolerance and hyperaccumulation of arsenic in plants by combining arsenate reductase and v-glutamylcysteine synthetase expression. *Nature Biotechnology*, 20: 1140–45, 2002.

259. Wagh, A.S., Huang, H.S., Hazardous waste, solidification and stabilization environmental analysis and remediation. *Encyclopedia Series*, 4: 2090–2102, 1998.

260. Basu, S., Wei, I.W., and King, P.H., Leaching potential of two industrial sludges: An evaluation of Toxicity Characteristic Leaching Potential (TCLP). In: *Proceedings of the 44th Industrial Waste Conference*, May 9, 10411, Purdue University, 581–590, 1989.

261. Trepanowski, J.J., Brayack, D.D., Nus Corporation, Devon, PA 19087 and Jeffery, A., Pike, V.S. EPA, Philadelphia, PA 1910. Investigation of stabilizing arsenic-bearing soils and wastes using cement casting and clay palletizing/sintering technologies, 1989.

262. Akhter, H., Butter, L.G., Cartledge, B.F.K. and Tittlebaum, M.E., Immobilization of As, Cd, Cr and Pb containing soils by using cement or pozzolanic

fixing agents. *Journal of Hazardous Materials*, 24: 145–155, 1990.

263. Trussel, S.A., Review of S/S interferences. *Waste Management*, 14(6): 507–519, 1994.

264. Twidwell, L.G., Plessas, K.O., Comba, P.G., and Dahpke, D.R., Removal of arsenic from wastewaters and stabilization of arsenic-bearing waste solids: Summary experimental studies. *Journal of Hazardous Material*, 36: 69–80, 1994.

265. Andres, A., Ortiz, I., Viguri, J.R. and Trabien, A., Long-term behavior of toxic materials in stabilized steel foundry dusts. *Journal of Hazardous Materials*, 40: 31–42, 1995.

266. Dutre, V. and Vandecasteele, C., Solidification, stabilization of arsenic containing waste: Leach test and behaviour of arsenic in the leachate. *Waste Management*, 15(1): 55–62, 1995.

267. Dutre, V. and Vandecasteele, C., Solidification, stabilization of arsenic containing waste from a copper refinery process. *Journal of Hazardous Materials*, 40: 55–68, 1995.

268. Buchler, P., Hanna, R.A., Akhter, A., Cartledge, B.F.K., and Tittlebaum, M.E., Solidification/stabilization of arsenic: Effects of arsenic speciation. *J. Env. Sci. Health*, 31(4): 747–754, 1996.

269. Akhter, H., Catrtledge, B.F.K., Roy, A., and Tittebaum, M.E., Solidification/stabilization of arsenic salts. Effects of long cure times. *Journal of Hazardous Materials*, 52: 247–264, 1997.

270. NEERI Annual Report 2004–05, P. 55–56. NEERI report on immobilization, solidification, and containment of arsenic bearing waste of Zuari Industies Ltd., Goa, 2005.

271. Pande, S.P., Deshpande, L.S. and Kaul, S.N., Laboratory and field assessment of arsenic testing field kits in Bangladesh and West Bengal, India. *Environmental Monitoring and Assessment*, 68(1): 1–18, 2001.

272. Deshpande, L.S. and Pande, S.P., Development of arsenic testing field kit: A tool for rapid on-site screening of arsenic contaminated water sources. *Environmental Monitoring and Assessment*, 101: 93–101, 2005.

273. Pande, S.P., Deshpande, L.S., Patni, P.M. and Lutade, S.L., Arsenic removal studies in some ground waters of West Bengal, India. *Journal of Environmental Science and Health*, A32(7): 1981–1987, 1997.

274. NEERI's Report entitled "Study of arsenic contamination in the ground waters of Block Chowki, District Rajnandgaon", submitted to PHED, Rajnandgaon Division, Madhya Pradesh, 2000.

Index